D0017353

issues

Coaching College Students

and

with AD/HD

answers

Patricia O. Quinn, M.D. ◆ Nancy A. Ratey, Ed.M., MCC ◆ Theresa L. Maitland, Ph.D.

ADVANTAGE BOOKS
1001 Spring Street
Suite 206
Silver Spring, MD 20910
1-888-238-8588

Advantage Books

Copyright © 2000 by Advantage Books

Library of Congress Cataloging-in-Publication Data

Quinn, Patricia O.
Coaching college students with AD/HD: issues and answers/
Patricia O. Quinn, Nancy A. Ratey, Theresa L. Maitland.
p.   cm.
Includes bibliographical references.
ISBN 0-9660366-7-0
1. Attention-deficit-disordered youth—Education (Higher)—
   United States.
2. Tutors and tutoring—United States.
3. Mentoring in education—United States.
I. Ratey, Nancy A., 1960–
II. Maitland, Theresa L., 1947–
III. Title.
LC4713.4.Q57 2000

The term AD/HD is used in this book in order to conform with current nomenclature. It is intended to include all aspects of the disorder, including non-hyperactive type, and is at times interchangeable with the terms ADD, ADHD, or ADD-H.

This book is designed as a guide to understanding AD/HD in college students: what it is, what it is not and ways to accomodate it in the college setting. The information is meant to enhance the reader's knowledge base; it is not meant to be used in place of formal medical diagnosis or appropriate medical treatment.

Published by
Advantage Books
1001 Spring Street, Suite 206
Silver Spring, MD 20910

10 9 8 7 6 5 4 3 2 1

Printed in the U.S.A.

Contents

To my husband, Joe, who has been my coach for many years.

To college students with AD/HD, as they struggle to achieve and live life on their own.

–POQ

To all my coaching clients: I dedicate this book to you! Thank you for asking me into your lives. I am forever grateful to have shared in your struggles and to have rejoiced in your successes.

To my father and Joe, and all the other "coaches" in my life: For helping me to believe in myself and to persist!

To my husband and step-daughter, Kath: For providing me with strength and hope.

–NAR

To my husband, George, for all the love and support he has provided and for bringing out the best in me.

To my parents, Joseph and Celia Laurie. I am grateful that I was blessed to have parents who had the God given ability to promote self-awareness and self-control in me, their most difficult child.

To Dr. Kimberly Abels for helping me find my voice as a writer.

To all the children, adolescents, college students and adults with AD/HD (and their families) who have shared their lives with me over the years, thanks for teaching me so much.

To Jane Byron and David Parker for the openness that allowed them to understand that college students with AD/HD had unique needs. Thank you both for having the courage and leadership to learn about coaching as a "better way" to meet the needs of college students with AD/HD.

–TLM

Foreword

AD/HD COACHING:
LOOKING BACK AND
LOOKING AHEAD

E ducational institutions at all levels are seeking ways to help students who are experiencing difficulty. There is a sea of change in progress and old ways are shifting, making room for the new. "One size fits all," a premise that has informed the way students have been educated in traditional classrooms, is being examined. Educators are realizing that you can't teach all students the same way because they don't all learn the same way. Individual differences has become a hot topic.

Since antiquity, man has been fascinated by what has variously been called the soul, the mind, or the brain. Individually and collectively, we've sought to understand what makes us the individuals we are, each with a unique constellation of characteristics.

The gallery of time shows us different portraits of the quest for knowledge about the self. Phrenology, the study of configurations of the skull in an attempt to understand the inner dynamics of the individual, was popular for a while. Examining "the humors" was prevalent in Shakespeare's time. Early twentieth century culture gave us Freud's model of the id, ego, and superego; today we have brain mapping and the current genome project. Our study of individual differences continues today and is intimately linked with how we understand and value biological diversity.

In some aspects of the natural world, we understand that biological diversity is essential to a healthy planet:

- People need to eat a variety of foods to maintain health.

- Crops need to be rotated in order to retain soil productivity.

- First-degree relatives are proscribed from marrying to ensure the genetic diversity of the species.

Yet we seem to have less understanding about how structural and/or functional diversity among individuals is consistent with this model. While we have learned enough about biological diversity to mourn the loss of a plant or animal species, we encourage and reward uniformity in people, and mock, fear, and reject differences. While in one realm we may have learned lessons about the necessity for diversity from disasters like the Irish potato famine, in the human realm we may be ignoring those lessons, and selecting for extinction divergent learning, processing, and thinking styles which have produced individuals like Thomas Edison, Leonardo da Vinci, Winston Churchill, and several Kennedys.

As we enter the new millennium, we need to take seriously the study of individual differences and to help students reach their potential, whatever that may be. We can no longer tell people they must learn a particular way. Rather, we need to discover how they learn and assist them in creating strategies and interventions that will benefit their learning process. And we must remember that learning does not come just from books, lectures, or laboratories. The most profound learning is often the result of a relationship over time that supports and encourages the process of learning—a relationship with a family member, teacher, trainer, mentor. Or coach.

Although "coaching" is a buzzword these days, it did not appear out of nowhere. In many fields including academia, the arts, business, and sports, a relationship-based association between individuals has existed dating back to antiquity. In some fields, one individual has paid another for his expertise and experience. In other fields, such as education, one person may be paid by an institution to provide instruction to other individuals. And in still different fields, no money is exchanged as one person assumes a role almost like that of a parent/guardian, guiding the other individual in matters that may include moral and ethical issues.

These coaching associations have existed in many fields throughout time. However, the first specific citation for AD/HD coaching is found in Hallowell and Ratey's book, *Driven to Distraction*, where on page 226 they bring AD/HD coaching into public awareness.

"What is an AD/HD coach? . . . an individual standing on the sidelines with a whistle around his or her neck barking out encouragement, directions, and reminders to the player in the game? The coach can be a pain in the neck . . . dogging the player to stay alert, in the game: the coach can be a source of solace when the player feels ready to give up. Mainly, the coach keeps the player focused on the task at hand and offers encouragement along the way. The coach can stave off a reversion to old habits of procrastination, disorganization, and negative thinking. Treatment begins with hope, with a jump-start of the heart. A coach . . . can holler at the AD/HD mind when it starts down the old negative grooves and bring it back to a positive place."

Coaching has evolved since 1994 when *Driven to Distraction* was published, but it is still always done in keeping with Hallowell and Ratey's original intent—to provide "hope" to the often-beleaguered individual with AD/HD. Hope comes as the client and coach work together learning how to manage the client's AD/HD symptoms.

ADD coaching is concerned with the practical matters in life—time management, organizational skills, memory problems, and any other functional difficulties an individual may be experiencing. It is holistic in approach. Coaching recognizes that a client is not just a student with academic concerns, but an individual who needs to eat nutritious foods to fuel his brain, get an adequate amount of sleep to function well, and remember to take the medication he has been prescribed.

Coaching is about keeping the student engaged in the process, learning what motivates him, helping him deal with procrastination, difficulty initiating an activity, and distractions. Coaching helps develop the needed tools, techniques, strategies, and interventions. Coaching encourages accountability and provides methods for reporting what has or hasn't been accomplished. Coaching develops trust in the process, the relationship, and the eventual outcome. Some people think we would all be lucky to have a coach!

Ultimately coaching is a vehicle for helping individuals become successful, according to their own definition of "success"—an admirable goal for any educational institution, whether it be Hatboro Elementary School or Harvard University.

Sue Sussmann, M.Ed., MCC
American Coaching Association
August 2000

Getting Oriented

AD/HD coaching as a field is taking shape rapidly. The demand for qualified coaches is increasing even faster. The purpose of **Coaching College Students with AD/HD** is to introduce those aspects of coaching that pertain specifically to helping college students with AD/HD make the changes needed to have a successful and balanced college experience. This book is not a manual on how to be a coach. It is meant rather to assist coaches, as they form a relationship with students with AD/HD who are attending college, and to help professionals who are not coaches, begin the process of understanding how coaching can be used with this population. Hopefully, this book will whet the appetite and encourage professionals to pursue more training in order to integrate coaching into their work with college students with AD/HD.

Part I of this book, **Introduction to the Coaching Model**, discusses some of the unique challenges faced by these college students as they transition to college. The concept of AD/HD coaching as a method to minimize these challenges and promote personal growth and academic success is also presented. Additionally, this section explores the theoretical underpinnings of AD/HD coaching and highlights those specific coaching tools and techniques that have been found to be effective in working with the AD/HD college population.

In Part II, **Issues and Answers**, the coaching process is brought to life by targeting and defining specific issues students with AD/HD commonly experience, and by offering a variety of coaching strategies that can be used to address these issues. In reading the suggestions listed in this section, it is important to keep in mind that coaching is a dynamic process driven by a client's individual needs, desires, and learning preferences. The power of coaching lies in the interaction between the coach and the client; therefore, the strategies presented need to be customized to the specific student and the situation at hand. It is important for the reader to remember that all strategies are ultimately worked out with the full involvement and consent of each student being coached. Hopefully, this section will provide insight into some of the causes of these problems, increase understanding as to how coaching techniques can be applied, and illustrate how coaching works in these cases. It is also the purpose of this section, to offer an array of concrete and tangible strategies that practitioners can use or modify to address particular issues with students with AD/HD when they arise.

Although coaching tools and techniques found to be effective in working with the AD/HD college population are being shared, this book is in no way meant to be a substitute for formalized training in coaching. For this purpose, individuals and organizations that provide training in coaching have been provided in the resource section of this book.

PART
I

INTRODUCTION
TO THE
COACHING
MODEL

Chapter one

Why Is College So Difficult for Students with AD/HD?

Jeffrey: A Typical AD/HD College Story

Jeffery is a first semester freshman at a local state university. He has agreed with his parents' suggestion to place a call to an AD/HD coach in the community near his university to see if her services could benefit him. The events leading up to this phone call are much more serious than the typical college adjustment problems that many students face during the difficult transition from the safety and structure of a family and high school to the freedom of college. Just yesterday, Jeffrey and his parents received his interim semester grades and, to put it mildly, "all hell broke loose." This young man, who ranked in the top fifth percentile of his high school class and excelled in Advanced Placement courses, is now in danger of flunking out of college. His parents drove in to visit him last night and took him to dinner to have a serious discussion about the terrible news they received. Jeffrey didn't need their stern looks and comments to make him face the significance of the grades on the report. He has known secretly how poorly he's been doing and has been in a state of depression for the past week or so.

From the start of the semester, Jeffrey experienced great difficulty juggling his academic work with the many social opportunities available to him on campus. He also quickly discovered that he could not keep track of the irregular class schedule he had at college where he had to attend different classes on different days. So, inadvertently, he missed a number of classes where attendance counted. Worse yet, he didn't know how to manage the volumes of daily, ungraded work he was assigned. He had never faced the situation in high school where work was not handed in, yet, he was expected to continue doing it on his own until the exam that would test his knowledge. When he realized that midterms were approaching, he tried frantically to catch up on all the reading he hadn't completed and to review all the notes he had taken. Unfortunately, he hadn't planned for the fact that his exams would occur within a two-day period. So, fatigued and stressed, he tried to stay up all night for as long as he could to cram. When he took the exams, his anxiety, coupled with the lack of sleep and inadequate preparation, caused him to misread questions and make many careless errors. For the past week and a half, since his exams, he's missed classes and stayed in bed most of the day. In the evening, he's gone out drinking with his friends, just to blot out his worry. He has felt nearly suffocated with anxiety about what his parents' reaction will be when they find out the truth. Finally, at the suggestion of the dorm resident assistant, he went to the university counseling center for help to cope with his emotional state.

How did this happen? Could this crisis have been avoided so both Jeffrey and his family did not have to endure the stress and frustration they are now encountering? Jeffrey was diagnosed with Attention Deficit Hyperactivity Disorder (AD/HD) in fourth grade, but he and his parents mistakenly thought it was no longer a major issue in his life. He excelled in a small high school without the use of medication and with hardly any support at home from his parents. Consequently, they all assumed that Jeffrey's experiences in college would be very positive. Unfortunately, no one predicted the host of new skills, supports, and structures Jeffrey would have to put into place to be successful in the complex environment of a college setting.

Jeffrey's parents hadn't realized how different the expectations he faced in high school were from those he would face in college. His high school had small classes where teachers took a personal interest in him. Jeffrey had also received the specialized services of a resource teacher, who worked with him to stay on top of his assignments and worked with his teachers to modify their expectations. Long-term papers and projects were broken down into small assignments that he handed in to his teachers throughout the semester. If he had trouble finishing an assignment, he could get an extension and then work with the classroom or resource teacher to complete the task. Because of his great verbal skills, Jeffrey really never had to research new information from his texts or other resource books. He could listen in class and use the Internet to do research for the few papers he had to write. His tests occurred every two weeks and he was forced to stay current in most classes because his teachers collected and graded his homework daily. Since he knew his teachers very well, they all gave him reminders about important dates. Because of all of this support, Jeffrey didn't really have to develop a system to remind himself about when things were due. Perhaps, Jeffrey's college disaster could have been avoided if everyone had a better understanding of how AD/HD was going to impact Jeffrey in college, and if Jeffrey could have been helped to develop the skills he needed to transition more smoothly into college.

While Jeffrey's case represents a combination of several real-life situations, the authors have observed many similar scenarios in their work with college students with AD/HD. The number of students with AD/HD attending college in this country has risen dramatically in the past decade. While few empirical studies exist to document this trend, available figures suggest that between 1996 and 1998 there has been an average increase of 52% (Parker, 1998) in the number of eligible students with AD/HD who are seeking help at college disabilities services offices. This figure does not include students who may have been diagnosed with AD/HD in childhood and, like Jeffrey, have erroneously presumed that it was no longer a problem, and have chosen not to disclose their disability upon admission. As Jeffrey's story demonstrates, these bright, creative students, their parents, and the professionals working with them have learned an important lesson: success in college for many students with AD/HD is similar to the task of mixing oil and water. The two don't easily blend together.

Why is college so difficult for individuals with AD/HD?

Success in college is dependent on a number of prerequisite skills that don't come naturally to individuals with AD/HD. College students must develop the ability to juggle competing social and academic demands and to independently form daily routines for waking up, bedtime, eating, studying, doing laundry, and other chores. They must also have acquired the strategies needed to complete long-term papers and projects, to conquer the voluminous reading assignments, and to prepare for infrequent tests with little or no external structure from instructors.

Although many college students with AD/HD have above average intellectual capacity and advanced academic skills, the symptoms of AD/HD can seriously limit them from demonstrating their full potential in college. Difficulty focusing and sustaining attention during writing tasks, a tendency to be easily distracted by more motivating and stimulating activities, and weaknesses in problem-solving skills needed to make decisions and exert self-control are common consequences of AD/HD. As Jeffrey discovered, if college students with this disability do not understand how these symptoms affect their lives and have not developed the tools necessary to manage them, they may "hit bottom" for the first time in a college setting. In fact, college is when many students with AD/HD are initially diagnosed because of significant academic difficulties or even academic failure. It is not uncommon for college students with AD/HD to experience serious social, emotional, and physical problems as they attempt to manage new expectations without the support and structure they relied upon in high school. Unfortunately, our entire society suffers when talented individuals with AD/HD do not achieve success in college.

While most colleges provide services for students with disabilities, these programs often are not a good match for students like Jeffrey. While some students with AD/HD may need tutoring because they have gaps in their academic skills, or notetakers because they have trouble listening in a large lecture, these services do not address the basic problem that Jeffrey experienced forming routines and developing a schedule to keep up with his work.

Likewise, most colleges have learning centers that provide services on various strategies for completing academic tasks like reading a text, writing a paper, or studying for a test. Such strategies have been used for years to help students with diagnosed learning disabilities (LD) and are the foundation of many college disability programs across the country. While these services may prove valuable for teaching students with LD, they may not be helpful for college students with AD/HD. In fact, the sequential process used to teach learning and study strategies to students with LD may actually bore the student with AD/HD who does not have a learning disability. Many students with AD/HD may be able to generate their own strategies or generalize a new strategy from a mere discussion. Their problems appear to be not in knowing what to do, but in getting it done.

Oftentimes, college students with AD/HD indicate that they do not need individual or group sessions on how to complete a task or how to better manage their time. As one student emphatically stated, "I know how to read my book and write my paper. I have taken every workshop my parents could find on these subjects. I can make a semester calendar and even use a day planner . . . I know how to plan. My problem is very simple; I just don't follow my plans. I need help making sure that I do what I say I am going to do, instead of procrastinating and getting sidetracked by other things. It would help me if I could check in with someone during the week to make sure I am on top of my work."

The unique problems faced by college students with AD/HD have created a need for professionals who work with them to develop services targeted to address these performance difficulties. While most college service providers and/or counselors may be comfortable meeting the needs of the students they encounter, they frequently discover that they are unprepared for the challenge of working with AD/HD students. Not only are their needs different from those of students with other disabilities, but they can have much more difficulty simply showing up for scheduled appointments or being on time to meetings. It is not uncommon for the student with AD/HD to really want to meet with a professional, but totally lose track of time and miss an appointment.

During these meetings, the professional may be overwhelmed by the communication problems some AD/HD college students exhibit. The student may set an agenda for the meeting and then spend the entire meeting digressing about some other less relevant issue. Problems in paying attention and effectively listening, as well as memory deficits, may cause the student to return a week later without having implemented any of the plans discussed or, worse yet, with no recollection of what was covered the previous week.

Professionals without an accurate understanding of AD/HD may immediately assume that the students lack true motivation to change. Even the most informed professional might not have the tools to deal with the differing needs and challenging behavioral patterns that AD/HD students exhibit. In an attempt to help students, professionals may provide unwanted feedback or offer strategies that inadvertently focus on the wrong issue.

Additionally, some college students with AD/HD may have negative attitudes about seeking help. They may still be struggling with acceptance of their disability and may be resistant to forming a working relationship with a professional. Some college students with AD/HD may have had a history of negative relationships with counselors or tutors who they perceive were foisted upon them by parents.

Many individuals with AD/HD are independent learners who admittedly do not learn through direct advice and prefer to handle things on their own. Seeking help can be even more difficult for students diagnosed late in adolescence who have absolutely no past experience with seeing a professional. These students have always been able to handle things on their own and getting help may be perceived by them as a sign of weakness or failure. As one college student with AD/HD declared when asked what it would take for her to seek help from a professional, "I would get help only if I could find a service that respected a willfully independent learner like me."

College students with AD/HD need a helping relationship that:

- Provides the support and structures that help them deal with performance problems caused by AD/HD.

- Allows them the freedom to design the relationship so they will remain committed to it.

- Allows them a comfortable setting to discover more about AD/HD and how it impacts their lives.

Coaching is the perfect relationship that meets all of these conditions and helps college students with AD/HD in a manner that traditional services do not. Hopefully, Jeffrey's relationship with a coach will help him experience academic success and allow him to demonstrate the potential he and his parents believe he has.

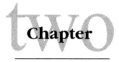

Chapter **two**

What is Coaching?

Coaching in sports

Today, we live in a world where we are surrounded by "professional trainers" and "coaches." We all have some idea of coaching from its use in the sports world. Individual athletes choose to work with coaches or trainers for very specific reasons. An athlete may possess a great deal of raw talent, but not be able to develop that talent to its maximum level unless a partnership is formed with a coach. Coaches are especially useful to provide encouragement, to give advice and constructive feedback, and to offer the motivation to overcome obstacles.

Coaches help the athlete generate and practice productive strategies for managing potentially problematic situations. Even when an athlete is discouraged, the coach pushes that athlete to continue towards his goal by training and preparing for the next big sporting event.

Looking at how coaching benefits individual athletes can help us begin to develop an understanding of using coaching as a model for working with individuals in other life situations.

Coaching can be seen as:

- A relationship that merges the potential for growth of the individual with the skills of the coach; as a result, the individual achieves more than he or she could have on his or her own.

- Facilitating the development and/or improvement of specific abilities and helping the individual achieve specific goals.

- Helping the individual by providing support, structure, supervision, and feedback before, during, and after performing the skills being worked on.

When the essential aspects of coaching are listed in this way, it becomes apparent that many of us have already assumed the role of coach, whether as parents, as mates, or with friends. In our professional lives, we may have also done some coaching as teachers, therapists, counselors, tutors, or learning strategy specialists.

The application of coaching to other fields

The coaching model has been adapted and applied beyond the sports world. Musicians, like athletes, use coaches to ensure that they create and follow rigorous practice schedules so as to develop their natural talents. In the business world, managers are being trained as coaches. Coaching is a novel approach to supervision, designed to bring out the best in each employee without using an authoritarian approach. In some situations, business coaches are peers who pair up with other employees to create a support system that promotes individual growth and productivity.

Recently, coaching has also evolved into a unique service that is being used to help any interested person improve his or her life. Many successful people hire coaches to help them take action on their dreams (painting, writing, gardening, exercising, etc.) and to achieve a greater sense of balance and fulfillment.

Personal and life coaching, as a distinct way of helping people, has its own philosophy and set of tools. Similar to sports coaches, these coaches attempt to draw out the existing talents and abilities of the person being coached. Personal and professional coaches presume that individuals have the power to recreate their own lives and the internal knowledge and resources to do so. It is the coach's role to provide the external supports and structures to help them focus on making the changes they choose. Following the implicit belief that the individual knows best, coaches seek input from the individual to determine how they want the coaching relationship to be structured and how they want the coach to respond.

Working with a life-coach allows individuals to be the "master of their fates" in the midst of today's hectic lifestyles. Life-coaches give their clients the opportunity to stop and take an inventory of their lives and design a new direction, instead of waiting for a major life crisis like an illness, death of a loved one, or tragic accident to provoke a change. Coaching, however, is not therapy or counseling, which helps the individual work through underlying emotional issues that are barriers to their happiness and well-being. Instead, life-coaches talk to people about action plans and how to reach their goals. Coaching creates a unique partnership, designed by the individual, that allows people to focus on their dreams and aspirations and to begin the process of taking the small steps to fulfill them.

Chapter three

Coaching for College Students with AD/HD

College students with AD/HD are typically bright, creative, and energetic individuals who possess enormous talents and aptitudes. Therefore, many find college a perfect match because of the freedom they experience, the challenging coursework, the opportunity to find outlets for their talents, and the fact that they do not have to sit all day like they did in high school. Some college students with AD/HD may have developed a keen understanding of their needs and the strategies necessary to be successful and actually flourish in this new environment. Others, however, may encounter great difficulty forming daily life and study routines, prioritizing the competing social and academic tasks, and using their time to get things done in an organized and timely fashion.

It may be harder for college students with AD/HD to focus, think before acting, stay organized, and monitor their attention and behavior over time.

Consequently, the college experiences of many students with AD/HD can be adversely affected by serious difficulties in time and task management caused by this disability. By forming a relationship with an AD/HD coach, a college student with AD/HD can be helped to develop the necessary routines and external supports needed to be successful. Coaching helps the student develop skills and strategies that allow him or her to compensate for areas of brain functioning which are affected by AD/HD. Coaching has been described as a perfect match for the AD/HD brain.

Experts in the field of AD/HD theorize that the problems one experiences in AD/HD are the result of differences in brain structure and function. The majority of research to date has shown an involvement of the frontal and prefrontal lobes of the brain and the areas to which they connect in the deeper parts of the brain (subcortical/striatal areas). These areas are specifically linked to motivation and emotional control—two brain functions that are adversely affected when a person has AD/HD. The executive functions of the brain, particularly attention, impulse control, goal orientation, and problem-solving behaviors, are all known to be dependent on the prefrontal lobes and their subcortical connections.

Without this executive control, a college student with AD/HD can experience great difficulty focusing and sustaining quality attention, thinking critically when developing a plan of action, having the self-control to follow through on the plan, and analyzing the effectiveness of the plan after it is implemented. Consequently, college students with AD/HD may not perform to the level of their abilities, in spite of their hard work.

College is, oftentimes, the first setting where many students with

AD/HD face the consequences of their disability. For some, initial diagnosis occurs when they "hit bottom" and for the first time experience academic failure and/or stress as they try to keep up with all the demands. In addition to needing strong academic skills, students must be able to monitor and control their attention and behavior. The college student must create and stick to a schedule that varies from day to day. In addition, there are a number of activities competing for the student's time and attention. These new demands for self-control occur simultaneously with a drastic decline in the amount of external structure provided. For many students, college is also the first time that no one is available to supervise them, remind or hold them accountable for getting things done. Now, they must literally think for themselves. While this independence may be a new experience for most college freshman, students with AD/HD frequently have little prior experience structuring their own lives and have relied on the external supports provided by parents and teachers.

Additionally, the academic demands of college escalate dramatically. In college, many students with AD/HD discover that their strong verbal and academic skills and sheer will power are not enough to pull them through. They must learn to face complex demands for independent learning, thinking more abstractly, and writing multiple, lengthy papers. There is often limited feedback on progress, since tests occur infrequently. A single project may be the basis of the entire course grade and homework is rarely collected and graded.

Without a well-developed mechanism to regulate, monitor, and control their attention and behavior, it's understandable why college students with AD/HD can experience significant failure and frustration as they attempt to plan, prioritize, and self-motivate. They often stay locked in a cycle of chronic procrastination. They have difficulty with initiation, and/or rush into action before identifying priorities and defining a plan to get things done in a logical fashion. Furthermore, AD/HD limits students' ability to use feedback and to engage in productive reflection necessary for learning from their previous mistakes. As a result, family members and friends who witness this repetitive cycle experience great distress. Many inadvertently become unwanted coaches giving unsolicited advice, reminders and help. Unfortunately, many students with AD/HD become frustrated, depressed, and stressed about their performance in college. Although they may know exactly what they need to do to improve their situation, they find it extremely difficult or even impossible to actually do what needs to be done.

Just as sports coaches help athletes reach their personal best, AD/HD coaches can provide the support, structure, and feedback needed to help students with AD/HD reach their potential. Using a model that is modified to the unique needs of college students with AD/HD, coaches facilitate the students' reflection, prioritizing, planning, and ability to follow a plan. Although the college student with AD/HD may resent the "nagging" and "help" of family and friends, they may realize that they can't navigate the confusing college landscape on their own. A coach can provide a more neutral, less-resented form of help. College students with AD/HD may, instead, choose to work with an AD/HD coach to deal with their difficulties. Over time, they can learn to motivate themselves, to plan more effectively, and to implement these plans.

The coach may be a professional working in a college learning disabilities program or as part of the university's counseling center. Some colleges have coaches as part of the academic skills program. The coach may also be working as a life-skills coach in private practice in the community and have experience working with college students with AD/HD. Regardless of the venue, the coach helps students with AD/HD develop habits that will promote academic success. However, the focus of the coaches' efforts may vary depending on the setting in which they are working.

The student's academic issues may be the primary focus if the coach is a professional working at a college or university. If the student has hired a private life coach, the focus may broaden to encompass all aspects of the student's life. Regardless of the parameters set for the coaching relationship, AD/HD coaching is a unique collaborative relationship that is designed to help college students with AD/HD develop the awareness, cognitive processes, behavioral patterns, and environmental structures needed to overcome the performance deficits caused by their disability.

A coach can help a student take action on his or her goals by working together to:

- Clearly define and prioritize realistic goals.
- Anticipate roadblocks that might prevent follow through on these goals.
- Develop strategies to address roadblocks.
- Create reminder systems to promote self-monitoring and improve follow through between sessions.
- Provide external accountability and evaluate progress toward these goals.

The coaching partnership allows students with AD/HD to learn the skills of self-management and self-motivation. By engineering their environment to become one that is AD/HD friendly, they learn to break the frustrating cycle of underachievement. With their coach, they learn to accept their AD/HD, to find out more about their brain, and to explore how they learn. Through this process, it is hoped that students with AD/HD will develop the strategies that will help them to compensate for weaknesses, to perform more consistently and to achieve academic success.

four

Chapter

Coaching: Getting Down to Business

A coaching scenario

During the first week of class, Lisa, a college student with AD/HD, attends a meeting with Tom, a college disabilities service provider and a trained coach. Lisa had a previous intake appointment during which she and Tom discussed her needs and goals, as well as the types of services and accommodations that are available from the center. Coaching was presented to Lisa as an optional service that Tom provides to help her stop procrastinating, a goal she has set for herself. Lisa decided to begin working with Tom in a coaching relationship. Let's join Lisa and Tom.

Lisa enters the office in a rushed manner and immediately begins to pull out folders, her daily planner, all her syllabi, and a legal pad from her backpack. As she piles her materials on the table in Tom's office, she begins speaking in an excited tone.

Lisa: *"I am feeling completely overwhelmed and it's only the third day of classes. All my courses have only two exams. What's worse, they all have these vague sounding major papers that aren't due until the end of the semester. This could be such a disaster for me! I love the classes and the concepts we discuss, but if I don't stay current with the readings and all these papers, I'll definitely have a major crisis at the end of this semester."*

Tom: *"It sounds like you are feeling pretty overwhelmed. It's so great that you decided to try our coaching services and that you made an appointment this early in the semester."*

Before reading on, stop and take a moment to write down or simply think about what your next step would be to help Lisa. With your approach clearly in mind, let's return to the meeting between Lisa and her coach.

Tom: *"Lisa, as I mentioned during our intake appointment, coaching is a partnership where you are in charge of what we do and how we do it. So, I'll need to ask you some questions during our meetings to get your opinion on a few things. First of all, what did you hope we would cover during our meeting today?"*

Lisa: *"Well, as I said, I am really feeling 'freaked out' by the fact that I have to stay on top of so many readings and about all the papers I have to write. I'm already feeling behind. I was hoping we'd spend time developing a schedule so I can begin working on all these assignments."*

Tom: *"OK, developing a schedule will be the focus of our meeting. Is there anything else you wanted to make sure we did today?"*

Lisa: *"Well, yes, I want advice on how to talk to my professors about AD/HD and the fact that I work with your center."*

Tom: *"So, you have two items for today's agenda. Well, Lisa, I also have some forms and procedures to go over with you about how we notify professors and decide upon accommodations. Let's see we have 50, no about 45 minutes now to be together today. What I have to do will take about 10 minutes. How should we divide the remaining time between your two agenda items?"*

Lisa: *"Actually, the more I think about it, I would rather use the entire time planning a study schedule. Can we postpone spending a lot of time on how to talk to my professors until next week?"*

Tom: *"Sure, I'll show you how we notify professors with our faculty letters today and, if you'd like, we can go into more depth on this next time."*

Lisa: *"Could you remind me that I wanted to talk about this subject when we meet next time? As you'll learn, there's no guarantee that I'll still be thinking about the same thing a week from now."*

Tom: *"OK, sure. Now, a couple more questions. Is there anything you want me to know about your preferences for communication and how AD/HD might affect you during our meetings?"*

Lisa: *"Definitely. As you probably already noticed, I can talk really fast and go on and on if I am stressed out about something or if I'm too excited."*

Tom: *"So, how can we handle it when this happens? Is there something I can do at these times that would be helpful?"*

Lisa: *"Just say something like, 'Let me interrupt here,' and* *repeat the question or say, 'Let's get back to whatever it was we were talking about.' Your comments will make me notice how I am feeling and help me calm down."*

Tom: *"Is there anything else you would like me to know about how AD/HD might affect our work?"*

Lisa: *"Yes, there's one more thing. If we make a plan for me to follow after I leave the meeting, I won't remember it if it isn't written down. So, let's stop the meeting a few minutes early and I can write down the plan in my notebook."*

Tom: (Tom records the procedures Lisa is requesting in her record for future reference.) *"OK, I think that's all I need to ask about right now, but I will be asking more questions as we work together to learn what your preferences are for how we should handle things. So, Lisa, what do you think would be the best way for you to make a schedule for yourself to get moving on your papers and your assignments this week?"*

Lisa: *"I think what I need to do first is to write down when each paper is due so I can see how much time I have."*

Tom: (Sits quietly as Lisa puts the paper due dates in her planner. When she's done, he speaks) *"OK, so how can you determine when is the best time for you do this week's reading assignments?"*

Lisa: *"I think it would help if I made a master schedule and looked at it when I have free time. Do you have a weekly schedule sheet that is broken down by the hour?"*

Tom: *"Yes, I do* (shows Lisa two different schedule sheets). *Which one of these might be best for you to use?"*

Lisa: *"I like this one because it goes until midnight and I don't really live a nine to five life. I want to go through and mark out all my classes, meetings, exercise times and meal times and when I usually sleep.* (She does this). *You know, there's a block of time every day right after class that would be perfect for me to do the readings.* (She highlights this with a marker.) *I would really like to try to get into the habit of using this time to work on my readings."*

Tom: *"Are you thinking that you would begin using that block of time for your readings today?"*

Lisa: *"Well, I suppose there is no reason to wait."*

Tom: *"What would it take to make this happen?"*

Lisa: *"I just need to go to the library and not go back to my dorm room. If I go back, I get tempted to hang out with my friends. If I can just make myself go to the library, I know that I will read."*

Tom: *"If you'd like, I can coach you on following through with doing your readings during that time today. For example, some students aren't confident that they will actually do what they say, so they want to check in with me in some way. They may choose to leave me a note reporting on their progress, or to email or call me to check in. It's important for you to know that this is an option and it is totally up to you if you want to be accountable in this way. Some students find reporting on their progress between appointments helpful, others do not."*

Lisa: *"I really think checking in would help me follow through. I am not sure about coming back here to write you a note, but since I check my email regularly, how about if I email you and tell you what I did?"*

Tom: *"OK, let me ask you a couple questions. If for some reason I don't get an email from you, should I contact you?"*

Lisa: *"Yes, definitely, because it means I forgot."*

Tom: *"What should I say in the email?"*

Lisa: *"Say, 'What's up? You were going to email me. Did you read today?'"*

Tom: *"So, if you did your readings during the time you wanted, what should I say?"*

Lisa: *"Don't make a big deal about it, just say, 'Great . . . so, how will you use tomorrow's time?' I hate when people make a big fuss over things I should have been doing all along. And if I didn't do what I planned, encourage me that changing will take time. Ask me to figure out what went wrong and how I can do better tomorrow."*

Tom: *"OK, I'll include those questions, and thanks for being so clear about what kind of feedback from me you will need."* (Tom and Lisa continue meeting.)

This quick look at a coaching session, should give you a general idea of AD/HD coaching and the issues that need to be addressed when working with college students.

The nuts and bolts of what an AD/HD coach does can be put into three basic categories:

1 AD/HD coaches explicitly **establish the procedures for the coaching relationship** or partnership to ensure a match to the individual's needs and preferences and to define the boundaries of the coach's role. Establishing the coaching relationship is much more than simply establishing rapport. During this process, the student "programs" the coach to get her needs met. You observed this when Tom deliberately inquired about Lisa's preferences for the meeting and asked for advice regarding how to handle Lisa's AD/HD when it impacted their conversations. He also found out what type of contact Lisa wanted between meetings and the precise type of feedback she preferred from him. By clarifying how Lisa could use his services, Tom is beginning to define his role.

2 AD/HD coaches **use questions** as the primary mode of communication to help guide self-exploration and to draw out the student's preferences, needs, and creative ability to solve problems. This is in line with how all life coaches work with clients and is based upon the belief that the person, not the coach, is the expert in the relationship. However, AD/HD coaches use questioning for another important reason—to help the college student with AD/HD engage in reflection and critical thinking that is difficult for him or her to do independently. The coach models how thoughts are used to regulate attention and behavior with hopes that the college student with AD/HD will eventually internalize this type of thinking. By posing questions, Tom helped Lisa become more engaged in solving the problems. Instead of reacting to her problems, Lisa was helped to reflect on how to best address them.

3 AD/HD coaches help students **develop internal and external structures** to focus priorities and develop an action plan. These structures allow the student to form new, more productive habits that promote academic success within the framework of a more balanced, satisfying life. Lisa and Tom are in the beginning stages of identifying some tools that will help Lisa manage her schedule: the calendar with paper due dates, the daily schedule, and emails to Tom about her progress. Because Lisa is selecting or creating these structures, there is a greater likelihood that she will actually use them.

In coaching, these three components are used deliberately and consistently to assist students with AD/HD in taking action on their goals and in learning about themselves. Coaching allows students to use their inner resources to identify and prioritize goals, to develop organized plans, to maintain consistent performance, to evaluate progress, and to develop self-awareness. Coaching is what happens when these components are blended together during a session.

The coach provides:

- External structure
- Accountability
- Feedback

As we stated previously, another unique aspect of coaching lies in the premise that the student, not the coach, is always viewed as the expert in the relationship. The coach becomes the student's partner as he or she learns to navigate the college experience. The coach helps students with AD/HD think before, during, and after they take the actions necessary to succeed in college. The coach is not acting in a traditional teaching or consultant role. For example, Tom didn't take charge of the meeting by deciding on the agenda or by selecting the type of calendar Lisa should use. He didn't automatically begin teaching Lisa how to manage her time. Instead, Tom drew out Lisa's viewpoints by posing questions to her. Although Tom may share suggestions, ultimately, it will be up to Lisa to determine what tools or external structures will be best to use in addressing her problems. Surprisingly, Tom and Lisa spent little or no time analyzing why Lisa procrastinated or focusing on Lisa's anxious feelings about all her work. Instead, he acknowledged her feelings and helped her move quickly into developing a plan to meet her goal.

You might be thinking, "So, what's new here? I always get input from students about what they want to do during our meetings and I also ask them questions to help them generate structures to use in their daily lives. I still don't understand what coaching is!" As you read the remaining sections of this chapter, you will discover the distinctiveness of the basic components of coaching and gain a better understanding of what a powerful intervention coaching is for working with college students with AD/HD.

Establishing the procedures for the relationship

As the scenario you've just read reveals, coaching is quite different from a traditional helping relationship in which the student is taught skills or strategies from an expert who assumes total responsibility for the session. Coaching also differs significantly from counseling or therapy sessions where the professional is helping the individual uncover and deal with the conscious or unconscious motives, reasons, or emotional issues that are blocking change or affecting happiness. The coaching relationship is a dynamic and powerful tool that is designed to bring about the **concrete actions** college students with AD/HD want to take by allowing them to tap into their own creative potential to reshape their lives.

As Lisa and Tom's interaction demonstrates, the procedures for the new relationship that develops between the coach and each student are explicitly "engineered" at the outset of the partnership. The Random House Webster's College Dictionary (1997) defines the word "engineered" in the following manner:

{**"Engineering is a process of designing to solve a problem."**}

This definition explains perfectly what was demonstrated in the scenario. To establish the relationship, Tom and Lisa designed a process to solve a specific problem by making decisions about what Lisa wanted to work on and how the coaching interactions would occur. These decisions are recorded so Tom can refer to them during future interactions. The coach and each student literally bring into existence a new relationship that is tailored to the preferences and needs of that particular student. As the student grows or new decisions are faced, the coaching relationship is redesigned.

Coaching is an ongoing dynamic process that changes and molds to the needs of the student as he learns about himself. As the scenario demonstrates, the coach does not make any assumptions about how or what to do that are based solely on past professional experience, observation of the student, or a review of the student's documentation. While the coach may use this information to suggest what might be the focus of the sessions or how the interaction might be structured, it is the student who is in the driver's seat and the professional who is the copilot.

This type of relationship empowers and motivates the student because he or she is truly "in charge." The collaborative nature of the coaching relationship is perfect for many AD/HD college students who have been independent learners with little or no prior experience working with a professional. Coaching can also dispel the fears of some students that the professional will take the place of parents, counselors, and friends who assumed the role of an "unwanted coach," nagging and reminding in a nonproductive manner. Coaching requires that the professional let go of the role of an expert or consultant and learn to share rather than to assume total responsibility for the coaching relationship. To be an effective coach, a professional must commit to adapting his or her typical style of working to match the diverse needs and preferences of each student he or she coaches.

To establish the relationship, the coach collects specific information from the student, both at the onset of the relationship and throughout its existence, in the following categories:

- The impact of AD/HD on the relationship.
- The student's patterns of past behavior.
- The student's preferences for feedback.
- The logistics and structure of the coaching sessions.

Impact of AD/HD

By asking the student how AD/HD impacts on the coaching work, the coach can quickly discover potential barriers to the success of the coaching relationship. In the previous scenario, Tom discovered immediately how Lisa's disability was going to affect their work and was given permission and guidance from Lisa on how to deal with things as they came up. It is not uncommon for college students with AD/HD to describe problems similar to Lisa's. Other typical responses include: difficulty attending or sitting still during lengthy meetings, trouble listening and following conversations in the sessions, being distracted by noises or visual stimuli in the office environment, difficulty remembering scheduled appointments, difficulty being on time to appointments and trouble remembering the plans developed during a session. Discussing these issues openly sets the tone for an *honest* relationship in which the consequences of the student's disability will be *understood rather than judged*. These discussions also prevent the professional from engaging in nonproductive speculation about the "whys" of a student's behavior and from becoming frustrated by nonproductive interactions with "difficult" students. When the coach is puzzled about how to handle a situation, he or she can simply ask the student for direction.

On occasion, college students with AD/HD may lack specific awareness of how AD/HD affects their communication or behavior. This is very common when a student is diagnosed late in life and is still adjusting to the news of having a disability. When the student cannot answer questions regarding the potential impact of his or her disability, the coach and the student can agree to learn together about the effect of AD/HD on the coaching relationship. In these instances, it may be helpful for a coach to describe patterns that other college students with AD/HD present in an attempt to help the student think about his or her needs. The coach and the student can choose a future date to summarize what is being learned and refine the relationship accordingly.

Patterns of behavior

It is also important for the coach to learn about behavior that the student has developed to cope with AD/HD. College students with AD/HD have a host of strengths to draw upon and productive strategies that have worked for them in the past. Conversely, they probably have also developed many nonproductive coping mechanisms that can be warning signs signaling a "slip" into ineffective coping mechanisms. The coach and student can agree up front on how to use information about positive and negative patterns. For example, the student may want the coach to build in reminders about a positive pattern at a time when he or she can't generate a plan. Similarly, the student may request that a coach ask periodically about the presence of old negative patterns and, therefore, help ward off a crisis. The following example from Tom's and Lisa's meeting shows how information about a student's pattern of behavior can be discussed.

Tom: *"Sometimes, when people are facing a crisis, they can become immobilized and forget how they have managed similar challenges in the past. Lisa, what are some of ways that you have successfully managed a crisis or difficult times in your life? If we have a list of the productive ways to cope, we can refer to these when challenges arise."*

Lisa: *"Well, one thing that really works, but that I hate to do, is to ask for help when I am stuck. I tend to feel that asking for help is a sign of weakness, so I avoid it. But every time I do, I can* *overcome the problem. I also do my best if I keep a structured schedule at these times."*

Tom: *"So, how can I help you remember to ask for help when you are stuck or to keep a structured schedule during a high stress time?"*

Lisa: *"I think you need to remind me if I don't think of these patterns. Lots of times, I slip back into the old habits and don't automatically think of what I know helps."*

Tom: *"It would also be helpful for us to be on the lookout for old negative patterns you've used in the past that spell trouble. What are these old patterns and what warning signs indicate that you are slipping into them?"*

Lisa: *"A major warning sign that I am slipping is the fact that I am late to appointments. Usually, I am late because I am staying up playing games on the computer or surfing the net."*

Tom: *"How would you like us to be on the lookout for these patterns?"*

Lisa: *"I think once a week you should ask me if I've been late to any classes or appointments."*

Tom: *"When we discover that this is happening what would you like me to say?"*

Lisa: *"It would be important to remind me that I told you this is a warning sign. Then help me think about what will happen if I keep this pattern going and encourage me to make a plan to change it."*

It can be useful for the coach and student to develop an ongoing list of productive and nonproductive patterns to summarize what the student is learning about his or her behavior. Since AD/HD can prevent students from reflecting and learning from the past, they can use the coaching relationship to facilitate this type of thinking. By doing so, these students are learning to engineer their environment to produce self-directed change and use the coach as an external monitor to help them remember and make it a habit. At predictable intervals (every month, at the end or the start of a new semester) the coach and student can agree to synthesize what they have learned.

Preferences for feedback

Another unique aspect of the coaching relationship involves the direct discussion about each student's preferences for how feedback should be given. As the scenarios with Lisa and Tom demonstrate, college students with AD/HD can guide their coaches to provide the exact type of feedback they need to remain focused during sessions, to critically observe their performance, and to remain motivated to achieve their goals. In the previous examples, Tom elicited this information by asking Lisa for clear guidelines on how to handle the times when her AD/HD is impacting her in a session or when her nonproductive behavior patterns surface.

Some students clearly want very direct feedback like Lisa requested if she changes a topic during a session or if she is late for appointments. However, some students indicate that a direct approach would not be helpful at all. These students tend to prefer that the coach use a more indirect approach to feedback such as posing questions rather than making statements. Some students indicate that indirect feedback lessens their defensive reactions, allowing them to process the information that is given. The following are some examples of indirect feedback: "Initially, you said you wanted to make a plan for your paper, now you are talking about your test. Do you want to change the focus of the meeting?" or "Is this an example of how you might change the topic?"

Students can also ensure that they get the type of feedback that keeps them motivated and helps them critically analyze their performance. When they have followed through on a plan, students can guide the coach on how best to respond. For some, too much praise is a turn-off, for others the lack of compliments would leave them feeling disappointed. Similarly, when a student doesn't follow through on a plan, he or she can guide the coach to respond in a helpful manner. Some students prefer to immediately reflect on what got in the way, while others want to postpone such reflection for fear of becoming depressed at their lack of action. They might prefer, instead, to simply go forward and define what steps will be taken immediately to compensate for the lack of follow through. Some students may guide the coach to ask questions that encourage them to face the possible consequences of not following a plan. Other students may indicate that no particular encouragement, questioning, or support from the coach may be needed; just knowing that they will be meeting regularly may provide enough structure and support to facilitate follow through.

The coach will be learning a lot about the student as they work together. Inevitably, he or she will have some feedback to share with the student. The coach can ask the student early in the relationship for advice on how such feedback can best be shared. Similarly, the coach can determine how comfortable the student will be giving feedback to the coach. Tom and Lisa address these issues in the example below.

Tom: *"Lisa, I have a few more questions to ask you about your preferences. As we work together, I will probably observe some things that I think might be beneficial to share with you about your patterns or how AD/HD might be impacting your performance. How might I best share this feedback with you?"*

Lisa: *"Personally, I would much rather you just say what you have noticed. I hate it when people beat around the bush."*

Tom: *"Similarly, how easy would it be for you to give me feed-back if there is something I am doing that isn't helpful?"*

Lisa: *"Well, now, that is a different story. I would find it hard to tell you something I don't like. Unless you ask me at the end of each meeting or after a few meetings if I have any feedback, I probably won't say what I am thinking."*

For many students like Lisa, giving feedback may be difficult. Students may indicate that a missed appointment may be a clue that something is "off the mark" in the coaching relationship. Politeness and a lack of assertiveness may prohibit many students from being direct. By discussing the importance of honesty in the coaching relationship, the student may become more comfortable about openly sharing their views.

Logistics and structure of the sessions and interaction

At the onset of their relationship, the coach and the college student with AD/HD need to clearly define when and how they will interact and what their mutual roles and responsibilities will be. Many college students expect the coach to tell them how often they need to meet or think that there is a right way to work together. It is imperative to impress upon the student that what is best for him or her is what will work. While the coach can share some options for how often interactions can occur, the student must be encouraged to agree to what he or she thinks will really be helpful. The student needs to determine the type of meetings and the frequency of contact that would be beneficial. The options may vary depending on whether the coach is in a private setting or in a college disabilities service program, but the following variations are possible.

- Shorter, more frequent, meetings to define immediate action plans instead of one longer meeting per week. For example, two half-hour contacts a week, or four 15-minute contacts a week may better match a student's needs. Or one lengthy meeting per week followed by daily email contact may help a student move to action.

- The use of email or the telephone for more frequent interaction may be beneficial instead of always relying on face-to-face contact.

- The potential for brief contact between coaching sessions to allow the student to report on progress or to be encouraged or reminded to follow the action plans developed during coaching sessions may be helpful. While some students may welcome the opportunity to be accountable and to be reminded, others may view this as similar to the unwanted nagging given by parents and friends.

Whatever the agreed upon arrangement, it is imperative to impress upon the student that the coach has no vested interest in a particular arrangement. For the coaching relationship to be effective, the college student with AD/HD must agree to a format that he or she is truly committed to and not one that simply "pleases" the coach.

The role of the coach on campus

As part of establishing the relationship, the coach's role needs to be defined so the student knows what to expect and understands the parameters of the relationship. College students with AD/HD need to understand that coaching is all about taking action on goals they set for themselves and developing the awareness, cognitive processes, behavioral patterns, and environmental structures needed to overcome the performance problems caused by AD/HD. Some students may say they want coaching, but they aren't really ready to share the details of their lives to be accountable to someone else or to make any changes. It is not uncommon for a coach to wear several hats as a disability service provider or as a counselor, therapist, or consultant. In such circumstances, it can be helpful to distinguish how coaching differs from the other roles the professional can play. Actually labeling the different roles as they occur might help the student sort out coaching from other services. For example, Tom might respond to Lisa in the following manner, "So, today instead of being coached you want to discuss accommodations for the tests you will be taking next week," or "It sounds like you are asking for some instruction in how to study for your exam."

While coaching is wholistic, the various constraints of college administrations make it impossible at most institutions for the focus to be this broad. The coach will need to explain that working on broader life issues, like paying bills, doing laundry, or developing an exercise routine will not be included as part of their work. Therefore, to uphold the wholistic nature of coaching, students being coached on campus may need to be referred to others to get their needs met.

The coach and the student also need to discuss how the coach will handle situations if coexisting issues outside of the coach's expertise continue to surface in a session. While the coaching relationship allows for the expression of feelings the student brings to the session, the coach can help the student identify when other coexisting conditions are truly blocking progress. At these times, the coach's role will be to encourage a referral to another professional such as a psychologist, psychiatrist, a counselor, or a substance abuse specialist. It may even be necessary for the coach and student to reevaluate whether coaching is really what is needed at a particular point in time. The boundaries of the coaching relationship will probably have to be reviewed periodically because the symptoms of AD/HD may cause students to be impulsive, forgetful, and to inadvertently continue to raise issues that are outside of the coach's domain. Open discussion of these issues can help prevent the student from feeling frustrated or rejected when the coach imposes limits, makes a referral, or redirects the discussion later in their relationship.

The use of questions as the primary mode of communication

Questioning is the primary mode of communication used in most models of personal and professional coaching and therapy. The questions coaches ask are designed to help the person take action by drawing upon their inner resources or to guide them in the right direction (towards their goals). Questions also help the person being coached learn about him or herself by prompting self-discovery. Coaching questions are quite unlike the questions asked in therapy that are designed to help individuals uncover their unconscious motives and analyze their past for nonproductive patterns of behavior. In coaching, the practice of posing questions is a direct outgrowth of the fundamental belief that the person being coached is the expert in the relationship. In fact, it may actually be helpful if the coach has no preconceived idea what the answers to questions might be. Then the conditions are set for the client to be the only source for the ideas that are generated. By asking rather than telling, the coach communicates the belief that the person "knows best." The coach is viewed, however, as a necessary partner helping the individual reach goals and make changes that are not possible without the coaching relationship. Certainly, coaches can and do offer advice and suggestions during a session, especially if the client doesn't take part in the solution. The bottom line is that the client decides whether or not to follow these suggestions.

Since it is assumed that the AD/HD brain is the main culprit preventing the student from implementing lasting changes, the coach uses questions to promote reflection and help college students with AD/HD focus, analyze, sequence, evaluate, and inhibit their actions. Questions prompt the use of the students' metacognitive ability— their higher-level thinking skills—that aren't easily mobilized when students with AD/HD attempt to engage in reflection independently. It is hoped that the students will eventually internalize these questions and become more proficient at this type of thinking.

The questions coaches usually ask fall into several categories.

- Questions to prompt short-term planning
- Questions to facilitate prioritizing
- Questions to facilitate follow through on a short-term plan
- Questions to promote self-observation and learning

In the following sections, more information is given on the purpose and types of questions a coach can ask in each of these areas. This list is not meant to be exhaustive, but to provide some suggestions on how a coach might use questioning while working with college students with AD/HD.

Questions to prompt short-term planning

While some college students with AD/HD are very skilled at planning and report that they don't need the coach for this activity, many indicate that they don't engage in effective planning. Their AD/HD brain prompts them to take action before having thought through the details of what they are going to do. For these students, an important function of coaching is to help them to reflect and define clear, realistic goals and detailed action plans that ensure success. The exact type of planning that occurs will depend on the student's preferences. As we saw in the scenario at the start of this chapter, Tom posed the following question to help Lisa develop a study schedule.

"What do you think would be the best way for you to make a schedule to get yourself moving on your papers and assignments this week?"

*"How can you determine when is the best time for you
to do this week's reading assignments?"*

These broad questions allowed Lisa to calm her emotions by focusing her creative ability on figuring out a plan to reach the goals
she set for herself. Once Lisa began to generate some ideas, Tom
posed the following question to help her apply her plan.

"What can you do today to begin using that block of time?"

Sometimes students come in with a less defined goal than the one
Lisa presented. They may say they want help in general planning,
in developing a schedule, or establishing a study routine. When
students have such broad agendas, the type of questions posed
will need to be different from those Tom used when he coached
Lisa. A list of some planning questions are provided below.

*"What is the time period for which you would like to plan
during this meeting (one hour, an afternoon, an entire day,
two days)?"*

"What do you want to accomplish during this time?"

*"How much time is really available during this time period
for you to accomplish your goals?"*

*"What options do you have for using this time to
accomplish your goals?"*

"What are the small steps to completing these goals?"

*"How will you use the time available to complete
these goals?"*

"How long do you think it might take to do what you plan to do?"

"Is your plan realistic? Do you have enough time to do what you have planned? If not, what options do you have?"

"How will you remember these plans?"

"What system for recording your plans works best for you?"

Questions to facilitate prioritizing

Prioritizing is an important prerequisite in the development of an effective short-term plan. For many college students with AD/HD, prioritizing is a very difficult task, limiting their ability to engage in productive planning. Frequently, college students with AD/HD express frustration when asked what their priorities are, since their "to do" lists tend to be filled with everything that comes to their minds for a given time period. Prioritizing can be even more difficult when there are a lot of things due at one time, such as during midterms and finals, if the student has procrastinated at doing what was needed. At these times, students may feel like "everything is a priority" and complain that they are unable to determine priorities among the list of tasks. Because of the frequency with which these issues present themselves, questions to prompt prioritizing during the planning process are especially important. When a college student is not able to rank the tasks within a list, the coach can pose the following questions to prompt prioritizing.

"Which tasks absolutely have to be done next or today?"

Sometimes just asking this question helps the individual begin to prioritize. However, when prioritizing remains difficult, the following questions can be useful.

"Are there any unnecessary tasks on the list that would be nice to do or that you want to do but really don't have to be done right now?"

"What are the deadlines for completion of each of the tasks on your list?"

"Are there any tasks for which the order in which you do things matters?"

"Are there any tasks that will take longer and have a more immediate deadline than the others?"

"Would it be helpful to use a calendar or some other planning device so you can see how things might fit together? If so, what device best suits your needs?"

"Are all of the tasks ones that only you can complete or can others be involved in helping you (e.g. campus resource people, etc.)?"

Questions to facilitate following through on a short-term plan

Many students with AD/HD report that meeting with a coach and defining clear, prioritized short-term plans is all they need to ensure that they will follow through and do what they plan. On the other hand, some students indicate that planning is not enough. Their main difficulties lie elsewhere. For these individuals, the emphasis needs to be on helping them actually do what they say they want to do. Tom questioned Lisa about this issue when he asked her if she would like to have a way to report on her progress. She agreed and asked for email contact between meetings to help hold her accountable for following her plan. Tom's way of bringing this up to Lisa can be used as a model of questioning students about whether they need more coaching on actually following their plans. Here is how he dealt with the issue.

"If you'd like, I can coach you on following through with doing your readings during that time today. For example, some students aren't confident that they will actually do what they say, so they want to check in with me in some way rather than wait until our next meeting to report on progress. They may choose to leave me a note, or to email or call me to check in. Some students find reporting on progress between appointments helpful, while others don't feel it is necessary."

For some students with AD/HD, being held accountable for their action is a very sensitive issue. They may have had very negative experiences with parents, teachers, and friends who nagged them and offered unwanted coaching to get them to do what they had to do. Others may also feel uncomfortable about having to be reminded or held accountable. They are embarrassed that they can't do things on their own, even though they know these coaching techniques might help. When they discover that they will not be judged, but rather be helped to learn what worked and what didn't, they are typically open to this aspect of coaching.

Below are some other questions that can be used when students agree that they want to be coached to follow the short-term plans they have made.

"Do you feel confident that you will follow your plans, or would it help for us to think about ways to ensure that you will follow through on them?"

"What would help you follow your plan?"

"What might interfere with your following the plan?"

"What could you do to prevent these conditions from interfering with your ability to follow your plan?"

"Will you remember these ideas or would it help to have an external reminder?"

"What system of 'check in' would you prefer? (emailing, phoning, or writing me a note after you have completed your plan)?"

"If so, who will initiate the contact? What will be communicated? How should I respond if there is no follow through or if there is follow through? If no contact is received by a certain time, should I contact you?"

"Would it be helpful to use rewards to motivate you to follow through? If so, what might the rewards be and how will you provide them?"

"Would it be helpful if you reminded yourself of the consequences of not following through? If so, how will you do this?"

Questions to promote self-observation

It isn't uncommon for the college student with AD/HD to come to a meeting with new and pressing issues without ever evaluating how the previous plan did or didn't work out. Again, the tendency to remain in action or to avoid reflection limits the individual with AD/HD from analyzing progress and learning from the past. Another important role the coach can play is to encourage the student to stop and evaluate how things are going. The coach and the student might agree to spend time periodically to prompt this type of thinking. The questions listed below can be used to guide such evaluation.

"What are you learning about how AD/HD impacts your academic life?"

"What helps you achieve your academic goals?"

"What gets in your way or doesn't work?"

"How have you helped yourself get back on track?"

"What are you learning about your preferences for studying?"

"Is there a best time of day for you to work on a particular task?"

"Do you perform better if you work on one task at a time or if you vary the tasks that you do?"

In summary, questioning is an important tool that coaches use frequently. This tool, which is the foundation of the coaching model, is especially matched to the needs of AD/HD college students. By asking instead of telling, the coach not only reinforces the notion that the student knows best, but also promotes reflection and models the use of thinking to analyze, evaluate, plan, prioritize, and delay action. By modeling powerful questions the coach is helping the student become his or her own coach.

The development of structures to help the student take action

Perhaps you have tried to form a new habit, such as exercising, dieting, stopping smoking, or taking a new medication. If so, you know that to be successful you have to keep your mind focused on the new behaviors. Otherwise, the old, unwanted habits can take over, driving you to do what you don't want to do. Think about a time when you have been successful at forming a new habit, what did it take? Perhaps encouragement from others helped. You may have used some external structures, like notes, lists, pictures, charts or calendars to remind yourself to stick with your plan. Maybe you redesigned your schedule and environment to make doing the new behavior easier. You might have eliminated cigarettes or sweets from your home, or made sure you went to the gym before going home after work. You probably also developed some new thought patterns to help yourself take the steps toward a new habit. Thoughts like, "I'll feel better if I do this," or "I'll hate myself if I don't do this" provide the kick in the butt to help us exercise when we don't want to or to pass up an extra helping of food. Thoughts like these probably served as internal structures, reminding and motivating you to follow through on a new behavior. Whatever the new habit you tried to develop, wouldn't you agree that changing behavior is, indeed, very difficult to do?

For individuals with AD/HD, developing a new habit or routine is even more challenging than it is for the average person. The naturally spontaneous, distractible, divergent mind of individuals with AD/HD doesn't engage easily in the type of thinking that is needed to stay focused on the new behavior and to sustain their efforts through all the starts and stops that occur when a new habit is formed. Without having external and internal structures to guide their behaviors, college students with AD/HD can get locked into nonproductive habits that interfere with their academic success. The following quote demonstrates the importance of structures in the life of a college student with AD/HD.

> *"Before being coached, I spent my day either being blown about by whatever task caught my attention at the moment, or in periods of obsessive work to meet a deadline where nothing breaks my concentration—not even hunger or sleep. I never thought through what my priorities were, what deadlines were around the corner, and what would be the best way of structuring my time to get things done. I just began doing or avoided doing things without a lot of thought. Now life flows so much more calmly and I am more productive. I now have the habit of questioning myself at the start of the day just like my coach does: 'What really needs to get done today? Are there any pressing deadlines around the corner? How much time do I have available today? What schedule makes the most sense? How will I*

take care of myself?' I am learning to use reminders, calendars, clocks and timers, other people, and rewards to motivate and structure myself."

Many college students with AD/HD report engaging in a similar pattern of fluctuating between periods of "hyperfocus," when they are driven by a deadline, and periods of "drifting" or being "blown about," when they are not consciously determining what they will do in a day. Add to the mix the fact that the college student with AD/HD is usually encountering, for the first time, the total freedom and responsibility of creating his or her own routines, habits, and schedules within the complex environment of college, while still struggling with the consequences of AD/HD. It is easy to understand why a coaching relationship can be used to help the college student with AD/HD develop the structures that will lead to academic success and a more balanced overall approach to life. External and internal structures can serve the purpose of helping college students with AD/HD remain focused on the changes they want to make and help them to produce these new behaviors until they become solidified as habits.

Developing external structures

The coaching relationship

For some college students with AD/HD, coaching services may make the difference between success or failure as they adjust to the complex world of a college campus. The coaching relationship itself serves as an important external structure many college students with AD/HD need to focus on their goals and to find the encouragement and structure to sustain their efforts. Just knowing that they have to set a goal in the presence of their coach may provide enough structure to help them take action instead of "drifting" or losing track of time. This relationship can help students be more serious about their goals and feel more accountable because they know that they will have to face their coach and "fess up" about their progress.

For some students with AD/HD, the coach can be the catalyst to propel them into taking necessary action. Besides planning and reporting on progress, some students may benefit from actually doing what they need to do during the coaching session. Students can use their time to make the phone call, send the email, begin reading the assignment or writing the paper they are avoiding. Once they have gotten over the hurdle of procrastination, the coach and student can generate a plan to keep the action going. In this way, the coaching relationship can serve as an important external structure to help the student focus on and face the important tasks they are not doing.

Rewards and consequences to promote follow through

The coach can help students with AD/HD determine how to productively use rewards and consequences as a way to motivate themselves to initiate and sustain action. Some students may ask the coach to provide rewards and consequences during their sessions or within the coaching relationship. For example, one student who was having trouble getting to meetings on time wanted the coach to cancel a session if he was more than ten minutes late. Another student wanted the coach to keep a chart for each goal attained. Some students do not want the coach to use concrete rewards and consequences, rather they want the coach to provide words of praise and/or reminders of the consequences that will happen if the action isn't taken.

Some students may prefer to identify how they can structure themselves by using self-administered rewards and consequences to motivate and sustain their performance. The coach can encourage the student to think about how he or she might be able to use rewards for following through on an action plan and what consequences might be imposed if the plan isn't followed. For example, one student who was constantly sidetracked by the temptation of surfing the Internet, chose to design his work sessions as 50 minutes of work followed by ten minutes of play on the Internet. He used a timer to monitor his work and play periods. This structure served an important role in helping him to initiate working when he was avoiding it and forming a new habit. After several weeks of doing this, he decided that he didn't need to be so structured because he was confident that he would work and limit his playtime on the Internet. Another student designed a creative mobile on which she placed stickers for each task completed on the road to writing a long, difficult paper. The ways to use self-administered rewards are as varied as the students needs and preferences.

Students can also be helped to effectively use consequences. In too many cases, students are great at self-punishment through the use of negative, harsh self-statements, but don't know how to productively apply consequences or to remind themselves of the potential consequences for changing their plans. One student developed the habit of making up the work time she had lost by watching television by trading time within her schedule for making up time spent viewing TV instead of feeling terrible that she didn't do what she had planned. If she spent several hours watching a video, she reclaimed some of her time to do the work she had intended to do. Another student learned to prohibit herself from going out with friends unless she read the daily assignment for class. One creative student made a list of questions to prompt her thinking about the consequences that she would face if she impulsively changed her work plans for the day. These questions were written on small note cards, laminated and placed on her key ring. She would thumb through them whenever her keys were in her hand, helping her stop and think about any spontaneous change of plans she was considering.

Other people in the environment

The coach can help college students with AD/HD use the significant people in their lives, such as friends, study partners, roommates, and professors, to add the structure and support they need to form new habits. For example, one student told his roommate exactly what to say and what not to say if he was observed to be off-task or obviously procrastinating. This assertive approach to asking for what one needs can prevent friends and family members from adding to the problem by making comments that are not helpful. Many students with AD/HD indicate that they are more likely to be on-task when they study with someone because they won't let another person down. These students can learn to form study groups with classmates, and schedule regular meetings with professors to show progress on long-range assignments.

Engineering the environment

The coach can help the student learn to engineer his or her environment to compensate for the problems caused by AD/HD. This might involve consciously modifying or changing where the student studies to make sure the environment is matched to his or her attentional needs. Although many college students with AD/HD want to be able to work at home or in their apartment, they may discover that this is a nearly impossible task, given the distractions that are present. As Lisa indicated during her coaching session with Tom:

> **Lisa**: *"I just need to go to the library and not go back to my dorm room. If I go back I get tempted to hang out with my friends. If I can just make myself go to the library, I know that I will read."*

Students can be encouraged to experiment and learn what environmental conditions help and what conditions hinder their ability to study. By turning on the answering machine, playing background music, or removing clutter from their desks, students may discover that they can work at home. Other students may realize that they need to leave home and go to a public place, such as a quiet restaurant or coffee shop, to face work that is unpleasant to do. Sitting in an easy chair at a bookstore may help the student face the dreaded task of drafting a paper or memorizing terms. Yet others may realize that the quietest corner of the library helps them focus or that studying at the university's learning center works best because they feel more accountable.

Students can also discover how to engineer their schedule to match their peak times for study and concentration. While one student may focus better in the morning, another may need to save difficult work for late afternoon or the middle of the night. Learning the truth about one's attentional preferences, as well as one's limits, is important. For example, how long can the student really work before needing a break? Does the student work best doing one task at a time or juggling several competing tasks at a time? A coach can help a student collect and analyze this type of important information so the student can begin to structure his or her life more productively.

Tools for time management

Coaches can also help students with AD/HD determine what type of daily schedule and planning devices work for them. Some students will never use day planners nor find semester calendars to be particularly helpful. When students are encouraged to be creative and design what works for them, they will discover strategies their coaches never imagined. One student discovered that a large white board with a list of important tasks for the next week is what she needed. Other students have designed their own computerized daily, weekly, and monthly planning sheets. Some students work best from priority lists with no time schedules noted because pinning down a specific time creates pressure and guilt. Others feel that they need to have a daily schedule filled in with what they will be doing within each block of time. One creative young man devised a way to use an 8 1/2 x 11 sheet of notebook paper folded into eight equal sections as his planning tool. He labeled one eighth of the paper for each day and the remaining section for tasks due in the future. He carried it with him in his pocket and used it to plan, schedule events and appointments and to remind himself of important future tasks. He reported that it had the added advantage of only showing him one day at a time so he wasn't overwhelmed, yet still allowing him to keep track of the entire week.

Through the coaching relationship, college students with AD/HD can think of creative ways to use the "things" in their everyday environment to help them remember and monitor themselves. By setting clocks, alarms, and timers, students can ensure that they change tasks when they planned, take a break to eat, take medication, or simply be aware of time passing. There arc amazing new devices coming out each day that can provide external structures: programmable watches, palm-sized computers, organizers, answering machines and services, beepers, and so on, that can be used to prompt, remind, and schedule. Students who are technologically skilled can program their computers to flash reminders. Throughout the day, a student can send a voice mail or email message to remind him or herself about daily plans. In a spirit of creativity and hopefulness, coaches can prompt college students with AD/HD to take a fresh look at their daily lives and to develop personalized external structures that will assist them in developing new habits.

Developing internal structures

"If only I would stop and think!" "Where was my mind when I made that decision?" "I just don't think about the consequences of my actions!" "I block my progress by being distracted by all the emotions I have about the task!" "Sometimes I know that I tend to lie to myself and think that I have enough time to get things done, but other times I'm really not lying. I just don't accurately estimate time." "I have a really hard time just keeping my thoughts focused and remembering what I planned to do." "Once I finally get working I am like a butterfly. My mind just flits from task to task."

These are all real quotes from actual college students with AD/HD that reveal the serious problems that can happen because they lack consistent use of productive, internal thought processes needed to guide, change, and monitor their behavior. While the natural style of thinking of AD/HD individuals may be a gift for drawing conclusions, being creative, thinking quickly, and juggling multiple ideas at one time, it can cause difficulties when slow, narrowly focused, sequential thinking is required. The coaching relationship can allow college students with AD/HD to refine these thought processes that are not as easy for them to use.

Planning and prioritizing

Coaches can demonstrate how thoughts can be used effectively before, during, and after an action is taken. Some students may independently begin to use the questions modeled by their coaches. Other students may require a more deliberate approach to applying these thinking skills outside of the coaching relationship. One college student with AD/HD reported her experience when she tried to plan and prioritize on her own during a time when her coach was away.

> *"I sat on the floor in my apartment with all my planning tools and my books around me, but I was immobilized. Without you (the coach) asking me the right questions, I got frustrated and sidetracked when I tried to plan. We have to do something so I know what questions to ask myself. I want to be able to plan on my own and not always depend on you!"*

To help students like this one become more proficient at using their own thinking skills, the coach and student can decide to re-evaluate their relationship periodically to slowly give the student more and more responsibility for doing the thinking that is needed during sessions. If the student chooses, he or she can create a list of questions or prompts to facilitate planning, breaking down a complex task, or prioritize several tasks. During the coaching session, the student can use these prompts to practice in the presence of the coach. These visual reminders can also be posted in a prominent place in the student's environment, like a day planner, mirror, refrigerator, notebook, or computer screen. As a student develops the habit of using thoughts in this manner, he or she will be more likely to develop the internal structures needed to be more independent at thinking objectively and critically.

Self-observation and self-monitoring

Thoughts play an important role in self-observation and self-monitoring. It isn't uncommon for a college student with AD/HD to say things like, "I have no idea what I did yesterday." "I didn't do what I planned, but I really can't remember what got in my way." Such comments reveal the serious problem many college students with AD/HD have in using their thoughts to observe and monitor themselves. The coaching relationship can be used to help students learn to develop these thinking skills. By reporting on their progress between sessions, students will practice self-observation and monitoring. Also, students can design personalized methods to help them be more aware of time passing. Some ideas actually used by college students with AD/HD are listed below.

- Writing down the time a task is started and when it is completed.

- Keeping the daily plan/goals visible and periodically asking, "Am I doing what I need to do?"

- Setting an alarm to go off periodically to prompt monitoring by asking, "Am I doing what I am supposed to be doing?" "If not, is what I am doing a more valid task?" "How can I redirect myself to get back on my plan?" "What am I feeling (hungry, tired, bored . . .)?" "What can I do to deal with these feelings?"

- Use naturally occurring break times to prompt reflection on the above questions (change of classes, after lunch, start of a new task).

Problem-solving and decision-making skills

In a similar fashion, the coaching relationship can help a student use more productive decision-making and problem-solving skills. College students with AD/HD frequently report that their tendency to respond impulsively and "get into action" may prevent them from thinking through their options when making a decision or solving a problem. They may select a paper topic, drop a class, or confront a roommate or professor about a conflict before reflecting on the options or potential consequences of such actions. To break this habit, one student developed a worksheet to use when pondering decisions or problems. This worksheet served as an external structure to increase the chances that the student would use the internal thought process that forced thinking critically before taking action. Another student put a post-it note on the phone to remind himself to say. "Let me call you back" when he got the inevitable phone call inviting him to go out with friends. By calling the person back later, the student would have time to think through the implications of spontaneously changing gears and going out with friends. The coaching relationship can help students become more aware of their problem-solving and decision-making strategies and develop ways to improve them.

Positive self-talk

Similarly, coaching can help students learn to counteract the use of other nonproductive thought patterns they have acquired over the years. It is not unusual for all of us to have inaccurate, self-limiting, and defeating thought patterns that remain unconscious and can prevent us from forming new habits. College students with AD/HD may have a larger share of such thought patterns due to a chronic history of not meeting expectations they or others have had for their performance. "I should," "I can't," "I never," "I always," "I have to," along with "I'll do it later," "There's plenty of time," and "It shouldn't take too long" are all phrases that may signal the presence of thought patterns that can limit progress.

In his book, "Taming Your Gremlin: A Guide to Enjoying Yourself," Richard Carson talks about the gremlin whose mission is to make us feel bad and prevent us from being the happy, creative individual we were meant to be. Becoming aware of how the gremlin or negative thinking is affecting behavior can be the first step toward change and growth. A coach is in a perfect position to help college students with AD/HD be on the lookout for such thought patterns during sessions and as the students attempt to follow their plans. For example, one student became aware that she was avoiding doing a tedious task for a long-term project by thinking, "It will be so boring. I'll hate it!" Instead, she decided to use a thought pattern from her childhood that helped her face the doctor when she was sick and needed bad-tasting medicine or a painful shot. On her daily schedule she wrote the words, "You can drag out the pain and make it worse or take your medicine and feel better sooner."

This thought helped to prompt her to tackle the unpleasant task knowing that it wouldn't go away and could become even worse. At times, the negative self-talk a student has may be severe enough to warrant a referral to another professional to deal with these emotions and the past events that caused these patterns to develop.

Conclusion

Coaching is a unique and powerful helping relationship that promotes growth and independence for college students with AD/HD by helping them overcome the performance and self-management deficits caused by their disability. The fact that the student is in the driver's seat and establishes the relationship, including the goals and methods used, increases his or her commitment and motivation to the changes discussed. No one is telling the student what to do or imposing a strategy or plan for a change.

The use of questioning as a primary mode of communication

empowers the student and reinforces the belief that he or she has the knowledge to solve his or her own problems or to find the available resources when he or she may lack the skills or strategies required for a particular situation. The constant exposure to thought-provoking questions also helps the student learn to stop and think more critically about the actions that he or she intends to take. Initially, the coach may serve as the external structure monitoring the development of new habits, allowing the student to follow through on short-term goals and plans. Independence is promoted as the college student with AD/HD learns how to develop the external and internal structures long enough to ensure that habits are formed.

Coaching can help college students with AD/HD learn how to use and manage their AD/HD symptoms and achieve their academic goals in ways that traditional modes of intervention cannot. A quote from one college student with AD/HD sums up how coaching can change lives. This college senior received coaching during her last year at college when she was diagnosed with AD/HD after nearly flunking out of school, in spite of her gifted intellectual abilities.

"For me, coaching has been a lifesaver. It has allowed me to have the hope to believe that I can change and find ways to stop my AD/HD from nearly ruining my college experience and my life. I can hardly believe it, for the first time in my entire school career, I actually read all the assignments for my classes and turned in my work on time. In the past, I wanted to be able to do this and I would go to the bookstore and buy all my books, thinking that this semester was really going to be different. But then I would lose my motivation and get overwhelmed by all the assignments I had to do. I realize now that I didn't know how to plan and structure myself to do everything. Because I worked with my coach, I could relax and trust that I

wouldn't fall behind. At the meetings, I would look at my syllabi to see what was due and work at a plan to do it. My coach encouraged me when I needed it and gave me a kick in the butt when I needed that, too. She even helped me learn not to rely on her; I now know how to plan and schedule on my own. I guess the most important thing about what I got from coaching is: I know what I need to do so I can do my best, and for the first time in a long time, I believe in myself."

PART
II

ISSUES
AND
ANSWERS

five

Chapter

DAILY LIVING SKILLS— ISSUES FOR THE COLLEGE STUDENT

What is it all about?

Recent research has led to a clearer understanding about AD/HD, which is now commonly accepted as a disorder affecting the critical skills needed to control one's attention. With deficiencies in these important skills, the individual with AD/HD can experience significant difficulty doing what he or she needs to do on a regular basis. In fact, many college students with AD/HD complain that doing the same thing every day at the same time is nearly impossible for them. They tend to resist mundane routines and habits and seek out the spontaneous and unpredictable. Others report being sidetracked constantly by distracting thoughts, competing activities, or old habits of getting lost in details or being perfectionistic.

Thus, the inability to form a daily living routine has the potential to be one of the greatest obstacles to success in college for the AD/HD student. In the face of infrequent exams and a host of independently managed assignments, the college student with AD/HD is likely to get stuck in a cycle of chronic procrastination and periods of deadline-driven productivity. Some students report getting totally caught up in all the exciting social and nonacademic experiences offered on a college campus, yet report wanting desperately to form the habit of doing daily reading assignments and reviewing class notes. The seductiveness of the moment can lead them to impulsively abandon plans to do boring tasks. While some report being laid back and enjoying the times before the deadlines hit, others complain that they can't enjoy their nonacademic time because of a nagging feeling of guilt that reminds them that they should be studying. Others indicate that they have attempted to develop a plan for daily living only to be frustrated at their inability to follow it. Some say that distractibility and spontaneity causes them to scrap any plan in favor of more motivating activities. Others report being frustrated when they discover that the original chunk of time allotted for a particular task isn't enough and realize that they have limited ability to estimate how long something takes to get done. Finally, some report losing time because of how inefficiently they complete a task. Negative self-talk that promotes being perfectionistic can cause a person to get lost in details or to overfocus on doing only a part of a task perfectly while losing sight of the big picture. Whatever the specific reasons a college student has for being unable to create daily living routines and then implement them, most share a common desire to break their current nonproductive habits and form new ones.

How can coaching help?

By forming a relationship with a coach, college students with AD/HD can have a partner who will help them form good habits and put in place structures that will provide the support they need to get up on time, exercise, eat regularly, do laundry, study, and make it to class and appointments consistently. The coaching session can be a time to reflect on the student's schedule and to think through a plan to help the student figure out how to get it all done. A coach can help the college student develop a mental time map of very specific time goals for fitting in all the activities he or she wants to pursue in addition to attending classes and studying. The student and the coach can review the class schedule and analyze the attendance policies of each class to make sure the student is informed of the consequences for being late or missing class. Since the coach is a nonjudgmental partner helping the student reach his or her goals, the student can be accountable and face the truth about his or her performance patterns. The coach can promote productive-thinking and problem-solving. By asking the student to focus on what steps he or she can take to deal with each daily living task, the coach can help prevent the student from falling into the old nonproductive pattern of avoidance or being stuck in worry or self-punishment.

The coach can help the student:

Develop a plan. Making and keeping commitments with oneself is a difficult thing for many students with AD/HD. Lack of structure and constantly changing schedules seem to make it impossible to develop good living habits. The intentions are in the right place, but all too often, students lose track of their goals in the shuffle of academic life. In order to make daily living skills into good habits, students need to develop a clear-cut plan—including accountability for action or lack of action to a coach—to ensure that these habits becomes a part of their daily life. A coach can help students take action and make it become a reality.

Keep the plan in mind. This is the hardest struggle for students with AD/HD. The coach can help with reminders and accountability through coaching check-ins, but it is up to the student to devise his own methods to keep the plan in mind, and to see and track progress. Some students mark their plan in colored pencil on their calendars, then post the calendars in a very obvious place so they see them on a regular basis.

"Program" the coach. It is important for students with AD/HD to know what sidetracks them from sticking to their plan. A coach can encourage students to verbalize this and identify ways to keep motivated, focused, and true to their plan. For example, if a student has difficulty managing time, but never says "no" to anyone who needs help, the coach might remind him of this problem and have him practice saying "no" more often.

Create a win-win scenario. It is easy for the student to set himself up for failure by expecting too much, too soon. This only leads to quickly abandoning the plan. Planning ahead helps keep the focus on what needs to be done. "What would happen if something came up unexpectedly with one of your classes and you could not go to the gym to exercise or to the cafeteria for lunch?" To accommodate such situations, the coach can help set a contingency plan for each week. This allows for flexibility but still holds the student to a minimum acceptable standard.

Let completing short-term goals drive the plan. Possibly the most important thing for long-term success is to focus on reaching short-term goals and not on how to get there. For people with AD/HD, this is even more crucial because they so often march to the beat of a different drummer. Don't worry if the best-laid plans are broken—focus on the short-term goals.

Issue:

Improving time management

Understanding the Issue

Most individuals with AD/HD struggle with managing time and forming routines. As Russell Barkley states, "Through no fault of their own, it is time and the future that are nemeses of those with AD/HD." (Barkley, 1997). Additionally, Kathleen Nadeau points out that "chronic lateness heads the list of the complaints made about adults with AD/HD." (Nadeau, 1995). Because of the basic problems individuals with AD/HD have using their thoughts to exert control over their attention, impulses, and behavior, many college students with AD/HD struggle with getting to where they need to be often arriving late, if at all.

Simply trying to learn a new schedule during the first weeks of the semester can be a monumental task for college students with AD/HD. Most college students have different schedules for different days. On Monday, Wednesday, and Friday, there may be one schedule to learn and another schedule for Tuesdays and Thursdays. This reality, when added to the pervasive problem that the student may have paying attention to time passing, estimating time, and then making the necessary decisions to be on time, increases the likelihood of missing or being late to classes and other important appointments.

Addressing the Issue

- At the beginning of each semester make an appointment with your students to go over their schedules. Have the students make out a detailed master plan of how they will spend their time each day and week that semester.

Encourage them to mark discrete start and stop times for every activity (waking up, showering, going to class, eating, exercising, socializing, laundry, paying bills, etc.) This kind of detailed planning allows the brain to slow down, think through all time commitments, and helps students to see time more accurately. It is unrealistic to expect that students will actually follow these plans exactly, but setting the intention of how they will spend their time allows them to know where they are supposed to be and when. Suggest that they post this time template where they can see it daily in order to keep their routine in mind.

- Make goals "survival goals" by keeping deadlines at the forefront of the student's mind.

- Have the student post a semester long calendar by the computer or bedside that includes all classes and other scheduled activities.

- As their coach, keep a copy of this same calendar in the student's folder for reference during discussions with the student and remind them at each check-in about upcoming deadlines.

- Have the student verbalize his or her goals to others: roommates, friends, and the coach. Discussing these goals helps to consolidate the student's commitment to act on them. This also creates social pressure to actually do what he said he would do.

- Create accountability and structure by setting agreed-upon start and stop times to study or perform other tasks. Have the student check-in via email or phone message with the coach.

- Help the student map out plans. By knowing what they

have to do ahead of time, students can focus on completing an activity, rather than on decision-making.

- Encourage the student to be honest with himself. Suggest that he keep a log of his time or create a system where he checks off what he has accomplished. Go over this report during each check-in.

- Encourage the student to practice healthy living habits. If he doesn't eat right, exercise, or get enough sleep, his chances of following a study routine decreases exponentially! Make sure to have these as a coaching goals.

Issue:	Establishing routines, rituals, and good habits

Understanding the Issue

Establishing rituals and routines is challenging for anyone no matter what age, culture, or economic background. Countless books have been written on how to change old patterns of living and develop new, healthier ones. Everyone can relate to the repeated struggles of trying to start an exercise program. It is hard in the beginning, but with proper commitment, planning and persistence you arrive at the day when you no longer have to "think" consciously about exercising—it just happens and miraculously it becomes part of our daily lives.

Routines and rituals reduce stress by providing a sense of consistency and predictability to our hectic daily lives. They are important for beginning each day in a directed way, for putting closure to the end of the day, for creating a rhythm to each week, and for helping us to automate otherwise tedious tasks.

Establishing routines and rituals is a monumental task for persons with AD/HD. Generally speaking, it takes about six to eight weeks of consistently repeating a task or action before it becomes habit. The AD/HD brain is highly distractible and has poor short-term memory—abilities that are key to successful habit development. However, the consistency and predictability that routines and ritual can provide, helps the AD/HD brain to minimize decisions, to focus on priorities, and to maintain a healthier life style.

The ability to develop good habits and rituals is crucial to academic success, and can make the difference between success and failure for students with AD/HD. Students with AD/HD have enormous struggles establishing simple daily routines like sleeping, eating and studying. Peer pressure, lack of structure, frequent schedule changes, and living in group situations all interfere with developing good habits. Despite the best of intentions, students with AD/HD have difficulties with the initiation of tasks, as well as with following-through—abilities needed to develop habits for successful college life.

Addressing the Issue

The coach can help the student:

Create "space" for habits. Part of the formula for habit development is creating space for good habits and making them a priority in life. This means recognizing the benefits and pay-off habits play in a student's college career. The presence of the coach can help hold that space open to explore what habits the student needs to establish and what helps and hinders the growth of routines and rituals in his life. This process will enhance the student's self-knowledge and increase his understanding of how to develop habits.

Break down the plan into doable steps. The coach can help the student break down actions into doable chunks and develop sequences for routines. The coach can help delineate ways to start the routine, to self-check, measure and monitor progress.

Keep the goal alive. The coach provides the needed "memory" to establish habits. By holding the student's agenda, the goal is kept alive and vivid. The bond with the coach helps to create "good stress" or "good guilt" and helps for more consistent follow-through over time.

Provide accountability. A coach provides the needed accountability and consistency over time to make actions habits. With the added support, encouragement and reminders from the coach the student is able to maintain the vigilance needed until routines become more automatic.

Issue:

Getting to class on time

Understanding the Issue

Being able to follow a class schedule and get to class on time is a basic requirement for being successful in college. During their first few weeks of college, many freshmen may find it to be quite challenging to remember where to be at what time and, more importantly, to exert the self-control required to get to their classes on time, if at all. Class schedules are quite different in college from what they are in high school. In high school, the only thing a student needs to do is follow an already existing, consistent schedule. Once a high-school student wakes up and gets out the front door, he or she can just go on "automatic pilot" throughout the day. Although high school students may be confused about their schedules for the first few days of each semester, most quickly memorize the day's activities.

While it is likely that some high school students, both with and without AD/HD, still rely on parents for wake-up calls and reminders to get out of the house on time, most students probably master the skill of getting up each day in elementary school. Likewise, in some situations, students may be tempted to cut a class or to skip out of school, but for most college-bound students, the consequences for unexcused absences are strong enough to prevent them from giving in to any temptation to miss class. Once they are in college, however, all freshmen have to quickly adjust to the fact that many classes do not take attendance or have attendance policies, and that they are pretty much left to their own devices to decide whether to attend a class or not. Furthermore, all freshmen must instantly develop strategies to get themselves up and off to class on time, to memorize their schedules, and follow them without any external structures and supervision.

For many college students with AD/HD, their college experiences begin to fall apart because they just can't get themselves up and to classes on time. On some occasions, problems getting to class happen for other reasons related to AD/HD. For example, the student with AD/HD may have actually checked his or her daily planner and have clear intentions to get to class at 11:00. However, he or she may totally forget about time, becoming lost in "hyperfocus" working on an assignment, and then rush into class 15 minutes late in an agitated state.

At other times, lateness or missing a class may not be the result of forgetfulness or being sidetracked by a distraction. Instead, the student may have totally unrealistic expectations about how long it may take to get from the dorm room to the classroom and not factor in time for the journey itself. College students with AD/HD appear to chronically underestimate the time it really takes to get from point A to point B, or how long a task may take that they stop to do right before leaving for class. One college student with AD/HD describes an example of this by stating, "I have mastered the art of forgetting time. What I mean by this is—when you look at your watch and you have 15 minutes before class you say to yourself, 'I can work another 12 minutes on the paper, and have three minutes to get to the next class.' What I don't take into account is the fact that it really does take seven minutes to get across campus, two minutes to walk upstairs to the classroom and find a seat in the class of 200 students. So, it really takes 10 minutes not three. I just don't have a mental time map."

While students may own clocks, beepers, alarms, and other electronic devices to remind them of the time and their schedule, they may be unable to consistently remember to program these tools to provide the external cues and prompts needed to be on time. Worse yet, they may carelessly put the wrong time for the class or appointment in their schedule or electronic device and show up at the wrong time or even on the wrong day. Of course, occasionally, the college student with AD/HD may choose lateness. He or she may realize what time it is, know that it is time to leave for class, yet chooses not to depart. Instead, he or she may decide impulsively to talk with a friend or do some last minute task. Unfortunately, at the moment the quick decision is made, the student frequently fails to bring to mind the consequences of these choices. The feelings of total panic and stress running across campus or of complete humiliation walking through the classroom door don't seem to come to mind until it is too late. Consequently, college students with AD/HD may frequently appear rushed, unprepared, disorganized, unmotivated, and/or irresponsible because of not getting to classes or appointments on time. Most college students with AD/HD report feeling terribly upset with their pattern of being chronically late or missing class and are not casual about this habit at all. Instead, their feelings of self worth are adversely affected by their inability to stop this self-destructive cycle.

Problems and/or differences in the sleep patterns of college students with AD/HD can further prevent them from regularly attending classes and important appointments. While most college students and adolescents adopt the habit of being "night owls," the students with AD/HD may have long standing problems falling asleep, remaining asleep, and waking up that may be diagnosed as full blown sleep disorders. Without parents to nag about bedtime and to assist them in waking up, the college student with AD/HD may find him or herself experiencing significant problems getting to the first class or appointment of the day, no matter when it is scheduled.

Finally, class attendance problems can occur because the student is simply unable to sit still for the duration of the class. Sitting in a large lecture class for 50 to 95 minutes can be a major challenge for an individual who is hyperactive and struggles with just being still and listening. Students with this profile have reported absolutely hating to attend long, boring classes. They report that this negative feeling can lead to the pattern of avoiding such classes altogether and then feeling guilty that they haven't been attending. They may find themselves stuck in a vicious cycle that they are unable to break.

Addressing the Issue

For going to class or to an important appointment

Strategies related to problems waking up

Help the student explore ways to:

1 Develop external structures to assist in waking up.

Examples:
- Set two or three very loud alarms (or purchase vibrating alarms for deaf individuals) to wake him up.
- Ask a roommate to wake him and reward the roommate with dinner or a movie.
- Ask the dorm resident assistant for support in waking up.
- Hire an answering service to place wake-up calls each day.

2 Create a daily routine and stick to it.

Example:
- Define a bedtime that is reasonable so that he or she will not be tired in the morning. Encourage the student to try to stick to this time no matter what, even on weekends.

3 Engineer the environment.

Examples:
- Don't schedule classes or appointments too early to avoid the struggle with waking up.

- Schedule classes with friends who can support attendance.

4 Seek out the help of another professional when needed.

Examples:

- Encourage the student to see a physician to discuss sleep problems.

- If the student is taking medication, help him or her to keep a log of how sleep is affected by the medication.

> **Strategies related to getting sidetracked or spontaneously deciding to miss a class or an appointment**

Help the student explore ways to:

1 Develop external structures to be aware of time passing.

Example:

- Use electronic devices as reminders about classes or appointments. (Set an alarm and attach it to a memo/ note indicating the consequences of missing class or an important appointment).

2 Develop external structures by being accountable to the coach.

Example:

- Agree to provide daily reports to the coach about class attendance (for example, call and leave a voice-mail message or send an email when leaving for class).

3 Use a reward/consequence system for attending/missing class.

Examples:

- The student may agree to give a dollar to the coach for his or her favorite charity for every time class is missed, or put a dollar in a "mad money fund" for his or her own use when successfully attending class.

- Reward himself for attending boring, unmotivating classes with a positive activity right after class, like meeting a friend for a snack.

4 Develop internal structures or positive thoughts that help prompt going to class.

Example:

- Tie class attendance to the student's life vision (especially important for boring classes) and have some sort of visual reminder about this vision on the book and notebook for the class.

Strategies related to getting to class on time

Help the student explore ways to:

1 Become more aware of time passing.

Example:

- Time how long it really takes to get to class and log this information to review during coaching sessions.

2 Set very specific time goals based on these observations.

Example:

- Develop a very specific time schedule, such as: I need to get up by 9:00 and be dressed by 9:30, have breakfast finished by 9:45, and be out the door by 10:00 to make it to my 10:30 class.

3 Engineer the environment.

Examples:

- Have clocks and watches in clear view.

- Use electronic devices as reminders for when it is time to leave for class.

4 Develop external structures by being accountable.

Examples:

- Have a friend remind the student when it is time to leave or that the goal is getting to class on time.

- Report to the coach on a daily basis (through voice mail, email, notes) about progress.

5 Be more thoughtful when planning class schedules for each semester.

Example:

- Select a schedule that spaces out classes so the student isn't running from class to class.

◊ Experience indicates that it really helps when professors have clear attendance policies, and missing or being late to class affects the student's grade. A number of students have stated that they wish their early morning classes had a professor with a strict attendance policy. One student reported that the only time she was on time to a class is when the professor closed and locked the classroom door when class started.

◊ It also helps the student if the coach or service provider has a policy for missed appointments and discusses this in advance with the student.

Issue:	
	Studying

Understanding the Issue

One of the first challenges a new college student must face is the need to develop a study schedule and routine. Many entering freshmen feel insecure about their ability to establish such a routine given the lack of the consistent daily structure that they had in high school. High school has a predictable daily schedule that leaves little room for decision-making throughout the day. When school lets out, most students participate in after-school activities that provide additional structure, leaving the decision of when to study or do school work to a fairly limited period of time. The high school curriculum also promotes the development of a study routine because most classes assign, collect, and grade daily work, and tests occur at frequent intervals.

Furthermore, class sizes tend to be small and students have a harder time hiding in the back of the class when they are unprepared for class discussion. Additionally, parents and teachers play an important role in reminding the student about assignments, as well as, supervising them during busy times when it is important for the student to buckling down. However, once in college everything changes and the student must generate and then follow his or her own study routine. This is a difficult task for many reasons. The daily schedule of classes varies from day to day. Some classes follow a particular schedule for Monday, Wednesday, and Friday and others have a different schedule for Tuesdays and Thursdays. Some labs or recitations only meet one time a week for an extended period of time. Depending on how the student has designed his or her schedule, there may be large gaps of unstructured time during the day.

Ultimately, one of the most glaring differences from high school is the total lack of adult prompting and supervision encouraging the student to study. Couple this reality with the fact that many college instructors do not assign, collect, or grade daily work. Students are expected to be self-starters, managing their own progress at completing readings and other assignments, and be prepared for infrequent tests or assignments that may not be collected until the end of the semester. Consequently, the need for entering freshmen to develop and follow a study routine becomes readily apparent.

The coaching relationship can help the college student with AD/HD conquer the challenge of forming a study routine. During coaching sessions the student can be helped to develop a realistic plan for studying that accounts for the student's disability. Many students report trying to copy their nondisabled peers and study for long hours in the college library, in spite of the fact that these expectations may be totally mismatched with the student's disability. By responding to the questions posed by the coach, the student can uncover his or her study preferences—the time of day that is best for studying, the location, the actual length of time he or she can remain focused, and how to best structure a study schedule. Instead of creating a schedule that is based on the "shoulds" that the student has adopted after years of failing at this task, he or she can be helped to design a plan that really works. When the student has limited awareness of his or her study preferences or what the barriers are to following a plan, the coaching relationship can assist in the important task of self-observation. Similarly, the coach can help the student become better at predicting how much time is needed for a given activity by collecting information and feedback from daily life.

The coach can also be the cheerleader, supporting the student through the difficult task of forming a routine for studying. When necessary, the coach can give students the reality check that is needed to remind them about the consequences of getting behind in their work. With permission, the coach can help the student catch the old nonproductive habits before a study plan is totally sabotaged. The student can also choose to be accountable to the coach by agreeing to log actual study time. If the coach works at a college disability center or counseling center, the student can choose to put in time studying on site and being present for an agreed upon period of time. The coach can act as the external supervisor providing the structure and support the student determines is needed to actually follow the schedule that has been developed.

Addressing the Issue

The coach can help the student:

1 **Develop a realistic study plan.**

Examples:

- The student can create an ideal study schedule based on his or her study preferences. This plan can be recorded on a master calendar to be used to prompt daily planning.

- After trying to implement the plan, the coach can encourage the student to refine it to match his or her needs. Students can begin to discover when is the best time to complete different types of assignments, how much time they truly need, in what order to do their work, what type of breaks are needed, and how often.

2 **Engineer the environment to facilitate following the study plan.**

Examples:

- The coach can help the student analyze what modifications need to be made in the study environment to increase the likelihood that studying will occur. This may involve any number of modifications, like putting a "do not disturb" sign on the door, shutting off the phone, going to the library, studying at a local coffee shop, studying in a setting where no one is familiar, timing medication to study periods, using ear plugs, putting on classical music for background noise, not working at a computer that is connected to the Internet, etc. One student reported locking his pleasure reading materials in a friend's dorm room until the study period was over to avoid temptation.

- Encourage the student to find a study partner who will study at the same time the student does to increase the probability that the student will follow through. Many students report that they will be more likely to honor the commitment to study when others are involved.

3 **Establish the relationship by specifying what type of feedback the coach should provide when the plan is followed or is not followed.**

Example:
- Early in the relationship the student can program the coach by specifying what to say or do when the study plan is not followed.

4 **Develop external structures that promote following through on the study plan.**

Examples:
- Make the student accountable for reporting on study time actually completed.

- Have the student report on study progress to a friend. Tell the friend what to say if the plan isn't followed.

- Make a sign that reminds the student of the benefits of daily studying and post the sign in a visible location.

5 **Use rewards to encourage following a study plan.**

Example:

- Have the student intersperse rewarding activities after periods of studying.

6 **Promote self-understanding by helping uncover what factors interfere with following the study plan.**

Examples:

- Observe and discuss how the symptoms of AD/HD appear to be affecting the student's ability to follow the schedule.

- Label other coexisting psychological or physical conditions that appear to be further interfering with the student's ability to follow a schedule or form a routine, like sleep problems, depression, anxiety, drug or alcohol use. Refer the student to the appropriate professional to deal with these issues.

- Identify how the use or lack of use of prescribed medical interventions may be affecting the student's ability to follow a schedule. Help the student collect these observations to share with his or her physician.

7 **Promote the development of internal structures that facilitate implementing a study schedule.**

Examples:

- Work with the student to have him replace negative self-talk with questions to promote introspection:

  What interfered with your ability to follow the plan?

  How do the symptoms of AD/HD show up and interfere with following your study plan?

  What type of thinking led to getting off schedule?

- Have the student come up with self-talk that will

encourage him or her to think positively and do what is planned rather than veer from the plan.

Instead of thinking, "I hate reading this stuff," say "I know this is not fun to do, but I will be glad it is done and I will do better on the test next week if I read a little now."

■ Have the student identify questions that will promote implementing the plan:

"What is the price I will pay if I don't do this now?"

"What is the priority task I am supposed to be doing right now?" "Am I doing it?"

■ Develop messages that will keep the student centered on the priority task:

"This is not the time to clean my room, I have time to do that tomorrow."

"Remember, all I need to know for the paper is the big picture, so I don't need to keep researching for more details."

"This is only the first draft, it does not need perfect sentence structure and wording."

Issue:

Keeping track of things

Understanding the Issue

Being able to gather one's self quickly and efficiently, to locate papers, to recapture ideas, and to remember details are all important to minimizing confusion and stress in life. It is these basics for developing habits that will keep a person in the running for the career or relationship he or she wants—one free of frustration and blame over things like losing keys, wallets, or important company files. The ability to capture and act on one's ideas is often equated with how smart or organized a person is. The person who constantly forgets what he said, or what was told to him, is seen as not only irresponsible, but unmotivated. This can have negative professional and social ramifications. Needless to say, this type of outer and inner organization is a key to one's success—both in and out of school.

For people with AD/HD, keeping track of things, both ideas and concrete items like keys, is a Herculean task. Often, when students arrive at school, it is the first time that they have to keep track of things on their own. The stakes are higher and they no longer have the external structure of home. There are more distractions, and, if they have not previously developed routines and habits for performing tasks, they now feel overwhelmed. Many students become paralyzed in this situation and can do nothing at all. Frequently people with AD/HD try so hard not to forget that they are taken away from the moment—if it is a lecture, they space out and miss important information, or if they are having a conversation, they tune out and make their partner angry.

Addressing the Issue

The coach can help the student:

Work on the process of discovery. The coach can assist the student in discovering what works and what doesn't by soliciting information on what strategies have worked in the past to keep track of things. A lot can be learned this way. For example, maybe in their home there was a hook on which to hang keys right by the door and on entry into the house everyone placed keys there. Or perhaps, there was a bulletin board in the family room where family members posted notices and reminders. By collecting this type of information, some of the solutions will be obvious. Simply recreate the same situations at school.

Make it habit. The coach can help to make intentions become ingrained habits. This is done by reminding the student that he or she has difficulties in this area and warning him or her to be hypervigilant until the habit has been developed. Repetition, vigilance, and reminders are key.

Take the blame away. A coach can help lessen blame and shame by helping the student to look at the situation through a neurological lens instead of a moral one. The good news is that the brain can learn. It may take longer for the AD/HD student, but it is doable.

Sustain attention and motivation. The coach can partner with the student in developing creative, fun solutions. By making it more of a shared goal, the student is more likely to stay motivated. When it becomes a game or something challenging and fun, the student will hopefully become more conscious of where things are.

Keeping track of things physical

Example: Dorm keys

Strategies

- Ask students each time you talk with them "Where are your keys?"

- Have them do email check-ins, specifically to report on where their keys are.

- Make this fun and nonjudgmental, like the game "Where is Waldo?"

- Have them carry their keys around their neck on a rope (this is very popular now).

- Have them "program" their roommates and friends to ask, "Where are your keys?"

- Put a screen saver on their computer to scroll "IT IS 5:00! DO YOU KNOW WHERE YOUR KEYS ARE?"

- Find out what personal items they never lose, and have them keep the key in that same place.

- The Sharper Image has a key finder that you attach to your keys. When you clap, it beeps. Suggest the student purchase one.

- Set up a system of rewards. If they keep their keys for X number of days, they can do Y.

- Keep a visual/colorful chart posted in the room where they check-off "I have my key" so they can see their progress.

- Have a huge sign on their door that says, "Do I have my keys?" or make it in code—give their keys a name like "Fred." "Do I know where Fred is?"

- Have the student make a "home" for the key; put a hook on

the wall, purchase a nice tray or basket. Through coaching, encourage the student to always put in it in there.

Keeping track of things mental

Example: Remembering extraneous, yet important thoughts

Strategies

- Introduce students to the concept of developing a "parking lot" or a "home" in which to park/place thoughts until they can be acted on, delegated, or deleted. This can be a designated place in their daily planner or it can be a place in their wallet where they collect these "captured" thoughts. Have each student designate a time to then go back over them or to transcribe them on to a to-do list.

- Ingrain this habit through the coaching sessions by asking the student, "What do you have in your parking lot?"

- Explore using a variety of reminder systems, such as a voice organizer or calling their phone answering machine with reminders to themselves. ("Call Bob tonight").

Issue:

Doing laundry

Understanding the Issue

Many students arrive at college not having had to do their own laundry. Some students don't know how to go about doing it on their own. Although it is a simple task, it does take time and planning. If the student has not been accustomed to creating time for this task in his daily life, it can seem overwhelming. Yet, this simple task is an important life skill for a variety of reasons. Primarily having clean laundry is a matter of personal hygiene. But, in college where students share small dorm rooms and have limited "personal" space, it is easy to make enemies of roommates if dirty cloths are left strewn about the room for weeks on end. Most AD/HD students don't think about doing their dirty laundry until they run out of clothes or the laundry pile gets to an unbearable level. Only then, will they marshal their attention and run off and do a load or two.

Often, it was their mothers that became the "environmental cue" reminding them to pick up their dirty clothes and to wash them, or sounding alarms by saying "This is unacceptable!" Often, without this kind of monitor, doing laundry doesn't present to students with AD/HD as something that needs to be done on a regular basis.

Part of being a responsible adult and living harmoniously with others requires one to take the initiative to clean up after oneself. This not only shows respect for other people's living space, but also helps in developing good personal living habits. An organized, clutter-free environment is helpful, if not necessary, to minimize distractions and maintain a sense of order for students with AD/HD.

Doing laundry on a regular basis can be a difficult task, especially when this mundane detail seems so small compared to other deadlines and getting to classes. How does a coach help a student with AD/HD get into the habit of doing laundry?

Addressing the Issue

The coach can help the student:

Recognize the importance of it. The first step is to help the student recognize the benefits of doing his laundry on a regular basis. He won't run the risk of upsetting roommates, and he'll save time not having to search for hours for a clean pair of socks or underwear! Doing laundry is a part of life, and unless the student can afford to pay a laundry service, he or she will eventually have to be responsible for doing this task. By making it part of the coaching goals and having the student be held accountable weekly, it will become a habit.

Set personal standards. Decide what is acceptable and stand by these set standards. Devise a scale using the student's personal standards and what can be tolerated in the environment. What is acceptable? What is unacceptable? Have the student check-in with the coach weekly and report a standard number/level. If the level is below tolerable, help the student come up with an arrangement as to how he or she will lower the number and by when. For example: 1) good (does not need attention), 2) okay (level is okay, no action needed for a few days), 3) tolerable (needs action soon—designate a time and day for it), 4) bad (needs action within 24 hours), 5) intolerable (needs immediate action).

Designate a time and a place for it. Designate one day of the week as laundry day. Have the student mark it on his calendar and make an appointment with himself to do it. Do it in the same place and at the same time each week. Never skip a week, no matter what else seems more urgent. This will help in developing a routine and making it become a habit faster. Repetition, repetition, repetition!

Enlist a "no excuses allowed" attitude. Actively plan for it. Don't let the student get caught short due to lack of planning. Always keep laundry detergent in stock and if the machine uses quarters, have a plastic Tupperware container filled with them. Help the student remember that there are no excuses that will allow him to skip doing his laundry on the designated day. Make a sign that says, "Just do it!"

Make it fun! Let's face it, doing laundry is boring! So, make it as much fun as possible. Suggest that the student do it with a friend, listen to his favorite CD while waiting for the clothes to be washed, or eat some chocolate—anything to help make it more exciting and to help pass the time.

Use visual cues. Have the student post a note on top of the laundry basket that says, "DO LAUNDRY ON SUNDAY". This will help to keep it at the forefront of his or her mind. (This strategy worked so effectively for one law school student that when her fiancé visited for the weekend, he did the laundry thinking the note was written to him!)

Group it with another activity. Suggest the student make laundry time "dual-purposed"—couple it with another activity. This will increase the probability of it actually happening and also of making it a habit. For example, there are some students who review class notes while doing laundry, or who go for a jog while waiting for their clothes to dry. Other students actually see this as "down time"—time they can spend alone reflecting on how classes went that week, etc.

The ability to establish patterns of daily living, and successfully tending to details like keeping up with one's own laundry, can be empowering. If these habits are not developed early on, the inability to do them can eat away at the very core of a person's confidence and self-esteem. These issues are often the skeletons in the closets of students with AD/HD. The feelings of shame and the amount of energy that is drained by either trying to tend to, or feeling guilty about neglecting these daily life details is immense.

Issue:

Exercising

Understanding the Issue

Part of maintaining a balanced life in college includes eating right, getting enough sleep, and exercising on a regular basis. Most current research dealing with health, reports that exercise is crucial to the optimal functioning of the body and brain. Regular exercise improves one's overall mental and physical health by decreasing stress and increasing one's ability to focus and concentrate more fully. Exercise is especially important to persons with AD/HD in helping to activate the brain and reduce restlessness. A regular exercise program can also help add structure to each day and provide an opportunity to socialize.

Knowing intellectually that exercise is good for you and actually making it a habit are two separate issues. Establishing the goal is easy. Remembering the goal, sustaining the commitment, and following through on a regular basis are the difficult parts.

Today, more and more high school students are arriving at college with team sports backgrounds. This is great! However, the AD/HD student who does not go on to play on a team in college can experience difficulty exercising on his or her own without the structure of the team and mandatory practice schedules.

There are several different types of exercisers:
- The year-round exerciser is a student who is a serious athlete and who has played on teams regularly or who comes from a family that values and emphasizes exercise as part of daily life.

- The occasional exerciser who has participated in team sports or takes ski vacations with his family, etc.

- Then there is the student who has no interest in exercising—who has not played on teams due to awkwardness, etc.

No matter what the student's background or athletic ability, now is the time to take exercise seriously. Developing the habit of and engaging in a regular exercise program is a commitment and investment that must be made in order to maintain a healthy lifestyle. Living with AD/HD is stressful enough, so exercising is not even a matter of choice—it should be done as a preventative measure against the stresses encountered in academic and adult life.

Making a habit of exercise is hard for anyone—it is hard to motivate oneself when it is cold outside or when one is tired and stressed. Students with exercise backgrounds are at a slight advantage, as they at least have felt the benefits (physical and mental) of exercise and can envision how good they will feel afterwards. Those students who have not had the benefit of that feeling may find it extra hard to motivate themselves, but all is not lost. Often these students have the best of intentions, but never seem to get around to exercising. Something "more important" always comes up—a friend needs advice, an assignment needs reworking, etc. A coach can help set up a regular exercise program and find strategies to motivate the student to follow-through on a regular basis until it becomes habit.

Addressing the Issue

The coach can help the student:

Understand the benefits of exercise to the AD/HD brain. Understanding how important exercise is to the success of students with AD/HD is key to making it a reality. If they do not understand how urgent it is to maintain a regular exercise schedule, they simply will not make it a reality. Educate the student as to the benefits and most importantly, encourage him to experience them!

Make it part of a natural routine. The very first step is to have the student examine his weekly schedule and get a clear sense of what he is doing on a daily and weekly basis. A coach can help in this process by asking questions such as: "What obligations do you have other than classes?" "Do you have any recurring weekly commitments?" (This includes things like extracurricular activities, therapy, or doctor's appointments.) By literally mapping out what a typical week looks like, the student can see his time and isolate places where exercise can naturally fit into the schedule. Before dinner or first thing in the morning are common times that work well for most students. Mark this on the weekly schedule so that nothing else will take its place. What is most important is that the student set the intention and protect the space. This weekly schedule should be posted in a visible place to remind the student of his commitment.

Get involved and try something new. Until exercise becomes a natural part of his life, the student should be accountable to the coach to try something new each semester. The coach can encourage the student to: sign up for an exercise class each semester; try something new and different like yoga or T'ai Chi; join clubs that require him to be in shape (i.e. the mountain club or water rafting); join noncompetitive teams; or partake in intermural sports like crew or running groups.

Make it fun—get an exercise partner. It is always easier to do things in groups or with the help of a friend. Ultimately, the initiative must come from inside of the student to exercise, but until it does, encourage the student to find a partner to help motivate him. Have him take the initiative and post signs or notices saying "Tennis partner needed" or "Jogging partner wanted."

Keep track of his progress. It is easy to think you have done something because it is on your mind all the time. "Remember to exercise!

Remember to exercise!" Encourage the student to log each time he exercises on his calendar, that way he will have a record of his true progress. Make it simple. Marking each day he exercised with an "E" for "exercised." Have the student be accountable to the coach for the times and days he said he would exercise and discuss what he actually did do. This kind of monitoring will help maintain steady progress towards making this goal a reality.

Move towards the positive, not the negative. Everyone knows how good it feels after a productive exercise session. Encourage the student to keep this in mind by thinking how good he will feel after he has exercised. Use this good feeling to motivate him towards exercising. If the student wants to make exercise a life-long habit, it is important that he be motivated by the positive, and not by negative thought such as, "If I don't do this I am worthless."

Schedule exercise appointments with himself. If it is not scheduled, it simply won't happen! For most students the difficulty is that of time management rather than a psychological barrier to exercising. Establishing an exercise schedule is key. It is easy to think the desire to exercise alone will get him to the gym—it simply won't happen if he doesn't plan it. A coach can help the student create a realistic and tangible plan for exercising on a regular basis. Assign a day and time and it will become reality.

Be realistic. Many students get discouraged easily because they set their sights too high, so be realistic. It's hard for most students to make time to exercise, so start slowly and set up a win-win situation. Setting a goal to exercise for an hour each day, seven days a week, is just not going to happen overnight. This all-or-nothing approach is a recipe for discouragement and failure. (The coaching rule here is, "Take what you think you want, and divide it in half.")

A coach can help the student identify the minimum and maximum number of days he can realistically exercise given his academic schedule. Help the student set a goal that he will be able to obtain no matter what—for example, "I will exercise a minimum of 20 minutes one time and a maximum of two times per week." Chances are he will at least meet his minimum goal. For many people, this type of minimum-maximum strategy for exercise works very well and builds encouragement, so that they can work towards exercising 4-5 times per week.

Set short- and long-term goals. Keep the "big picture" in mind. Mark exercise goals on a calendar—for example, it might be to be exercising four/five times a week by the end of winter semester. This allows the student to see the overall goal with a timeline attached—three months to get up to speed. From there he can work backwards and develop goals for each month—two days per week in September, three in October, and finally four in November, etc.

Create a history of successes. The key to progress for the student is making it measurable and knowing what he did or did not do. This is a common struggle for students with AD/HD because they often lose track of activities done during the week. It all becomes a blur and often students feel that they have accomplished nothing. To alleviate this, a coach can help the student devise a calendar as a sort of "score card" to mark an "E-Y" ("Exercise-Yes") on the days that he does exercise and an "E-N" ("Exercise-No") on the days he does not. This way he can see his progress and monitor whether or not he is reaching weekly and monthly goals. It helps to create a history of successes. The key is to make it visible and simple.

Make it habit. This means doing it repeatedly over time—during vacation breaks or during exams, when the student needs it most for stress and concentration. Encourage the student not to skip— no matter what. Even 15 minutes is better than no exercise, and he will stay in the habit and create space for it.

Other strategies include:

Having the student

- Consider the time he has set aside to exercise as an appointment with himself.

- Enlist a "no excuses" attitude—if he catches himself thinking about whether to exercise or not, stop and simply walk out the door to the gym.

- Keep an extra gym bag packed with exercise gear in the car and in the dorm, always ready to go when he is.

- If finances allow it, hire a personal trainer to guide the workout.

- Remember that there is no tomorrow in NOW. Just do it!

- Visualize how good he will feel about himself after he has exercised.

- Know and understand what current research is saying about how important exercise is to the AD/HD brain.

- Understand that there are no failures—only those who give up. The AD/HD coaching motto is, "Fake it until you make it!"

```
Issue:

          Eating regularly
```

Understanding the Issue

Going off to college can pose many new challenges for students with AD/HD. Many of these challenges stem from the lack of structure in the university environment. In order to be successful, students need to be able to create their own structure. If not, simple daily routines, like eating meals on a regular basis, will be lost. Most students arriving at college have come from homes or settings where they never had to think about when, what, or where to eat—this was the responsibility of parents or other caretakers. At college, it becomes even more important to eat meals, not only for the social factor that meals can provide, but also to maintain good health habits.

Along with the lack of structure, students with AD/HD frequently skip meals because they aren't hungry. Many are taking medication that diminishes their appetite; therefore, they often simply forget to eat. Or worse, they will gorge or binge-eat late at night when their appetite returns.

Although most undergraduates live on or near campus and belong to meal plans, there are many who don't. This circumstance provides added challenges in that there is the extra time required to plan for and cook meals. A coach can help students be aware of their eating habits and can stress the importance and benefits of maintaining healthy eating habits.

Addressing the Issue

The coach can help the student:

Become accountable. Encourage students to report on meals as part of their check-in. Having them account for their eating habits can help to keep the importance of these habits at the forefront of their mind, and help them to establish the habit of not skipping meals.

Have meal times written into a schedule. Help students establish a ritual around eating, so they will anticipate meals times. Encourage them not to skip meals, even if they aren't hungry. For example, have them eat at the same times each day—morning, noon, and evening meals. Have them group the meals with other activities. For example, have them plan to eat breakfast after their shower every morning, or go to the cafeteria after their 11:00 class every day, etc.

Avoid binges. Even if a student reports to you that he or she only eats a small amount, stress the importance of eating something, and not skipping meals. Explain that otherwise he or she might be prone to binging late at night. This can not only cause weight gain, but also interrupt the sleep cycle.

Make eating have a social purpose. Brain storm ways to make meals fun with your students. Have them meet a friend, classmate, or faculty member for a meal on a regular basis. Help them make the meal and socializing part of their weekly routine. If a student lives off campus, have him or her get in the habit of sitting down for meals with roommates. You might also suggest making grocery shopping a group event. This will engage everyone in the process, and help make sit down meals more likely to happen.

Create self-awareness in the student and encourage him to plan ahead. If the student knows that he tends to skip meals, or gets hungry at odd times, help him put this information to use. Have him think of ways he can create a habit of carrying snack food with him. Have him be accountable for going to the grocery store on a regular basis to purchase healthy snack foods to help hold him until meal times.

Create an eating "smart" food attitude. Encourage the student to learn as much as he can about nutrition. Eating a variety of foods in the right combinations is essential to proper brain and body functioning. A diet of all carbohydrates will only leave him feeling hungry and depleted — he should also eat protein and foods high in fiber, nutrients, and vitamins. Create accountability or have him meet with a nutritionist, if more counseling is necessary.

◊ Eating disorders are common in the college population and may be more prevalent in students with AD/HD. Refer students to other professionals, if eating too much or too little appears to be a more serious concern.

◊ An excellent resource to address student's eating habits is Anne Selkowitz Litt's book, "The College Student's Guide to Eating Well on Campus," 2000, Bethesda, MD: Tulip Hill Press.

Issue:

Waking up and staying up

Understanding the Issue

Being able to wake-up and stay awake are dependent on having healthy living habits. Getting enough sleep, eating well, and exercising on a regular basis are essential to a healthy life style. Doing this however, takes organization, planning and vigilance on the part of the student so as not to get off track and loose sight of his academic goals (to get to class, to complete papers on time, etc.) as well.

A common struggle for students with AD/HD is not being able to "wake their brains up" in the morning. Many students complain of walking around in a "fog" and not being able to think straight. Having a clearly defined set of activities to do each morning helps the brain to focus in on priorities. Establishing morning and evening routines and rituals creates structure and minimizes the chances of getting lost in the morass of indecision that plagues students with AD/HD.

Routines and rituals serve to keep students with AD/HD more focused on their goals and deter them from being swayed to "goof off" with roommates or by other temptations in the environment.

Addressing the Issue

The coach can help the student:

Set a "bed time" alarm. Have the student set an alarm to "go to bed" to ensure he will get to bed at the established bed time.

Repeat the same sequence of activities each night and morning.
This is a very powerful tool to automate important actions that
need to be done (for example, looking at one's day-planner!) and
make them a habit. This can best be done by helping the student
to create evening "wind-down" and morning "wind-up" routines.

Example:

Evening "wind down" checklist:

- Clear desk top and put books in backpack.
- Look at day-planner for what is ahead for tomorrow.
- Review goals for that day-what ones remain?
- Make a "to do" list for the next day.
- Set out cloths to wear.
- Brush teeth.
- Set alarm.
- Set out medication beside alarm.
- Get into bed.

Morning "wind-up" checklist:

- Wake-up.
- Take meds.
- Check to-do list and goals for the day.
- Take shower.
- Dress.
- Go to breakfast.

Have the same wake up time each day. Through coaching, reinforce the habit of waking up at the same time each day and going to bed at the same time each night—no matter what time the student's first class is that semester! This helps to set his "internal" clock and makes waking up a lot easier.

Set up regular accountability checks. Have the student set up regular accountability and progress measures with the coach to make sure he is reaching agreed upon targets.

Set a wristwatch or use or a countdown timer that beeps every hour. By using a timer, the student can learn to group activities into "time segments" or "blocks." Example: wake-up, be out of bed, showered and out the door *in one hour.* This helps to "chunk" a series of activities together but also helps to create added "stimulation" to the situation. If the student spaces out and spend too much time in the shower, he can try to "beat the clock" by completing the rest of the checklist in 15 minutes instead of the planned 30 minutes. This also allows for some flexibility in completing the routines and can reduce boredom of doing the same sequence over and over again.

Arrange for an automatic morning check-in. Have the student check-in each morning with the coach upon waking or brainstorm other ways to be accountable and follow-through. For example, meet a classmate for breakfast each day. It is a lot harder to break a promise to someone else than it is to break one made to yourself!

Issue:

Getting to bed

Understanding the Issue

Possibly one of the most difficult challenges for an AD/HD college student is having a reasonable and regular bedtime. In order to do this, the student must first break the bad habit of staying up until early morning hours. In college, without the structure of their home environment, AD/HD students quickly forsake their evening goal of studying or getting to bed early to join dorm buddies in all night bull sessions or other spontaneous activities. Soon a pattern is established of staying up all night and sleeping all day. This is a sure formula for failure and is difficult to break. Many excuses are given by students for staying up until dawn: "It is quieter and I can study then." "It is the only time I have to myself and I want to relax by surfing the net or watching TV." Another popular excuse is: "In high school I did all my projects by pulling all nighters and got A's!" Students are caught off guard when their old high school strategies fail them in college. They end up paying the cost of waiting until the last minute, staying up all night in a panic and then missing classes to catch up on sleep.

To break these negative patterns and establish new healthy ones, the student must have a clear sense of the benefits of establishing regular bed times. Creating a habit of going to bed each night at a reasonable hour is key to success. Working with a coach can begin the process to stop these old destructive habits and replace them with new healthy ones. A rested student is more prepared to handle stress, learn new material, and use his time more efficiently. If the student does not believe this, he will continue to fool himself into thinking he does not need to have an established bed time.

Addressing the Issue

The coach can help the student:

Increase learning about and acceptance of one's brain. Help the student value the importance of learning as much as he can about his brain. Learning how to operate at the optimum level is the first step. Oftentimes, students with AD/HD have not taken stock of what helps or hinders their concentration or performance levels. When they reach college, they fool themselves into thinking that they are like everyone else and that it will not take that much of a toll on them if they pull some all-nighters or stay up late. Working with a coach can help them take the time to reflect on these issues and put up roadblocks so they don't keep following the same destructive path. Facing the truth is not always easy—but the truth is that the AD/HD brain is different. Help them to be honest with themselves about this. Help create some understanding around their limits. This is difficult to do, but it is part of the process of living and learning with an AD/HD brain. Warn them against fooling themselves into thinking it is simply a matter of willpower.

Effectively manage transitions. Students often complain of getting stuck on or sucked into projects. This tendency is as powerful as an addiction. Surfing the net for obscure details for a project or simply to escape for awhile can side track them for hours at a time, week after week. This can also happen with TV, talking to friends, etc. By being open and honest with the coach about these issues, a student can start to put plans in place to self-check these tendencies and create strategies that help him stop an activity and move on to the business of getting to bed. There are several strategies that can help him better manage this transition:

- Using environmental reminders. Using the environment effectively is a very valuable tool for persons with AD/HD, yet it is often overlooked. Doing simple things like having them agree to shut down their computer after 11 PM or posting a note to themselves ("Do not log on to the Internet after 10 PM") on the computer screen, or having a screen saver that scrolls the message "NO INTERNET AFTER 10 PM" are all strategies students have used successfully.

- Being conscious of choices. Part of stopping old habits is to become more conscious of them. A successful strategy used by one student was to put a towel over his TV. The act of removing the towel helped him to slow down and think long enough to stop before he turned on the TV. Becoming conscious of what he is about to do, can help the student make better choices and "talk" to him or herself about their actions and the inevitable consequences.

- Creating accountability. This can be done by suggesting that the student keep a score card of the times per week they have gotten to bed at their agreed upon times. This helps to keep the goal alive, and creates a means of measuring progress and celebrating wins. This same type of strategy can be used with friends and roommates. By verbalizing his goal and asking for their help in reminding him to "get to bed" if they see his light still on or they see him wandering the halls at 2 AM, the student is more likely to achieve his goal.

- Measuring time correctly. Part of transitioning from one activity to another involves correctly measuring time and "labeling" time with discrete activities that are to be done in each time block. For example, some students set an alarm to remind them to stop what they are doing and prepare for bed. Others set two alarms—one to remind them to stop one activity and then one set for 15 minutes later to help remind them to start to get ready for bed.

- Creating a distinct set of activities. Help students establish routines that they can follow, or create a series of activities to be done in a sequence each night. This is a powerful tool to help students transition from one activity to another, such as going to bed. Each activity should have a start and an end time to help create a sense of flow and to help them not get stuck (for example, spending one hour flossing their teeth because they decided on a whim they would try to do better than their dentist). Over a period of time, and with reinforcement from their coach, students will get into a habit of doing a sequence of discrete activities—one after the other. For example: brush teeth, put on PJ's, set alarm, review daily goals, put books in backpack for next day, write to-do list for the next day, go to bed. This will help automate the process and help the student wind down while they prepare for bed.

- Breaking down the problem. Of course, there may be other reasons why a student might stay up late. A coach can help the student explore some of these issues. For example, he might not have a problem getting to bed, but he may have difficulties falling asleep. This might be an issue that can be medicine-related. Or perhaps the student has found he cannot fall asleep because his environment is too noisy. Exploring different options, such as white noise machines, earplugs, or perhaps changing rooms, might be very helpful.

Also, if a student is staying up late as a way to study in a quiet environment or to get time to himself, then you as their coach can help him devise other ways of filling these needs during the day, so as to not interfere with the need for a good night's sleep.

Issue:

Taking medications

Understanding the Issue

Stimulants are the treatment of choice for AD/HD, but must be taken regularly to be effective. As students with AD/HD establish a more independent lifestyle, they inherit the task of becoming more responsible for the medical treatment of their AD/HD. This primarily involves taking stimulant medication, monitoring its effectiveness, and reporting or dealing with side effects. During the elementary and high school years, this responsibility usually fell to a parent who maintained contact with the prescribing physician, renewed prescriptions, and obtained refills. In addition, the supervising parent would monitor the student's compliance with the recommended dosing schedule by noting the number of pills consumed and the time between refills.

Compliance can often be an issue for high school students with AD/HD. They frequently stop taking medication during the school day because of the embarrassment or stigma associated with having to go to the school nurse or other personnel authorized by the school to obtain a mid-day dose. In addition, many students with AD/HD like how they feel when energized or hyperactive, and fall victim to the encouragement of friends who find them more entertaining or fun to be with when not taking medication that decreases hyperactive or impulsive behaviors. While some students may see the value of taking medication for study or homework, most have not come to appreciate the benefit of improved attention and focus during other activities such as athletics, driving a car, reading, or even more mundane tasks such as cleaning their rooms. Here the problem lies partly with the prescribing physician and other mental health professionals who frequently fail to perceive AD/HD as a quality of life issue and thus fail to educate the student about the benefits of taking medications for real-life situations other than school or academics.

High school also differs from college in that the high school day typically begins in the early morning and lasts until mid-afternoon. Freshman college students, therefore, do not have the experience of dealing with varying class schedules and the considerable free time during the day. If he does continue to take medication to improve attention and focus, the college student may not know how to schedule doses to achieve the desired result. For some students who did, however, find medication to be effective during high school, starting college exposes them to another huge pitfall. Students frequently equate leaving home and living independently as an opportunity to wipe the slate clean. They incorrectly assume that they now can do it on their own, and don't need the medication and other supports. They discontinue all treatment, failing to see that it was these very treatments that generated the success resulting in their getting into college in the first place. These students, frequently, don't realize the trap that they are setting for themselves until it is too late in the semester and they are substantially behind in class assignments and seriously placing their grades and college standing in jeopardy. It is only then that they seek the help of a coach.

Addressing the Issue

The coach can help the student:

Increase awareness. First, and foremost, the coach needs to discuss with the student the purpose of taking medication and what he or she has experienced as specific benefits from taking this particular medication. How is the medication addressing his or her primary symptoms? With the help of the coach the student may also need to develop increased awareness of how AD/HD impacts all aspects of daily life and to determine which situations he or she wants to improve by taking medication.

Set up a schedule. Remembering to take medications is very difficult under any circumstance. AD/HD affects an individual's ability to remember and to follow routines. Therefore, students with AD/HD will need assistance from the coach in forming a routine to take medication consistently. Brainstorming to determine what is getting in the way, and setting up a medication schedule with built in reminders and supports will be of utmost importance.

Establish reminders. Merely setting up a schedule for taking medications, however, may not be enough. The student obviously needs to remember to actually take the recommended dose of medication. Students often ironically complain that they forget to take the pill that is going to help them to be better at remembering. By devising a system of reminders, the coach can assist the student in reaching the goal of actually taking medications on a set schedule. More importantly, a system can be developed for taking medication for an activity that may not be part of the student's daily routine, but is one in which medication would clearly enhance performance.

Monitor effectiveness and side effects. Students frequently take medication, but lack a systematic method to evaluate its effectiveness or to report side effects that may arise. One goal of the coaching process could be to set up such a system. This would include isolating target symptoms and routinely quantifying how taking the medication reduces or eliminates them. Having the student complete a checklist at regular intervals is an effective way to help monitor the occurrence of side effects. Role-playing can also be used to help the student become more comfortable in relaying these side effects or other concerns to his or her physician.

Obtain refills. Most college students continue to rely on their hometown pediatrician or psychiatrist and obtain their AD/HD medication refills from home. This usually consists of placing a call home and asking that a new prescription be obtained and mailed to them at school. Because of their AD/HD and the inability to adequately plan ahead, this arrangement often results in the medications arriving after the prescription has run out. In addition, the student does not see or talk with the prescribing physician directly and therefore, no one is attending to compliance, appropriate dosing schedule, effectiveness of dose, or side effects. The coach can definitely be of assistance here by encouraging the student to take responsibility for his or her medication management and to pursue transferring the process for renewing prescriptions to the campus health center or a local physician or psychiatrist. This arrangement also provides a greater opportunity for face-to-face assessments with improved monitoring and discussion of issues.

Store medication. Over the years stimulants have been used inappropriately by some college students who have abused controlled substances. College students with AD/HD have reported having their stimulant medications stolen because they are not carefully stored. Other students have shared stories of being badgered by students without AD/HD who wanted to buy pills to improve attention and enhance studying for tests or exams.

In addition, some students with AD/HD report that their own disorganization has caused them to lose their pills, only to discover that their doctor would not refill a prescription. The coach can help the student avoid these problems by discussing ways to safely store medication.

Strategies for dealing with medication issues:

- Ask about the use of medication during initial meetings with a new student and periodically with former students. "What is your understanding of how your medication works?" "Are you taking your medication consistently?" "When you take it, what have you noticed?"

- If your observations suggest that a student is not taking his or her medication, share your concerns about this." I'm noticing that you seem to be having trouble concentrating today, I'm wondering what's different today? Have you taken your medication recently?"

- If you discover that the student has questions or concerns about medication that are interfering with using it, suggest that he or she contact the prescribing physician. You may need to facilitate this by helping the student list the questions, plan a time to call, role-play the conversation, and/or make the call or write an email during a session.

- If the student is not taking medication because of forgetfulness or disorganization, ask if he or she would like to spend some time during the session developing a plan to remember his or her medication. If the answer is no, keep the door open for a future discussion when the student might be more interested.

- Determine if the student has been able to remember his medication at other times or has developed other important routines. Analyze what has helped in the past and list these for future reference.

- If the answer is yes, involve the student in developing a plan to remember to take his or her medication.

- Discuss with the student newer longer-acting preparations of stimulants that last 8 to 12 hours. These preparations may eliminate the need for several doses per day. The student should be encouraged to discuss these medications with his or her prescribing physician.

Developing a plan for taking medications

Define the problem:	■ I keep forgetting to take three doses of medication a day.
Assess factors contributing to the problem:	■ I wake up too late to pack up my pills. ■ I don't pay attention to time.
Brainstorm options:	■ I could pack my pills the night before. ■ I could wake up a half hour earlier. ■ I could set an alarm watch. ■ I could ask my girlfriend to remind me. Remember to draw on past success— what worked?
Evaluate options:	■ I won't get up early. ■ My girlfriend isn't in all of my classes.
Select the best option and define a plan for it:	■ I will pack my pills the night before, when I set my alarm for the morning. ■ I will set my alarm watch for the second and third doses.
Determine the type of support the student needs to remember to follow the plan:	■ How will the student remember? *Post-it-Notes on the refrigerator and mirror.* ■ What might interfere? *I might not be able to find my pill bottle.* ■ Would the student like the coach to act as an external support as he or she forms this habit? *Email? Frequent check-ins? Phone contact?*
Evaluate the implementation of the plan:	■ Be prepared for limited success. ■ If needed, use steps one through six to revise the plan.

Chapter Six

SOCIAL SKILLS— ISSUES FOR COLLEGE STUDENTS WITH AD/HD

What is it all about?

What is it? What does it help with?

The expectation for most 18-year-olds, today, is that by the time they graduate high school, they have automatically become adults. This means behaving accordingly—being responsible, mature, and articulate. The ability to get along with others, make a good first impression, engage in small chat, abide by social norms, listen attentively to others, and maintain eye contact during conversations can determine the success and direction of one's professional life. These same "social skills" also impact one's personal life. College can be a perfect venue for most young adults to develop socially. Living in group situations, relating to peers whose background and culture is different from one's own, exploring and defining one's own sexuality, and interacting with faculty, staff, and university personnel all add to the richly diverse social experiences encountered in college. During these crucial developmental years, young adults can spread their wings, shed old "stereotypes," and develop a new sense of self and create their own identity. Because of the importance of social skills to life beyond college, some academic institutions are teaching social skills as a way of better preparing young adults for the world of work. The Massachusetts Institute of Technology's "charm school" helps students learn how to negotiate the intricacies of social interactions, and some business school programs are including table manners and appropriate dress as part of their curriculum.

College can either be a rewarding or a challenging place to develop social skills for the student with AD/HD. Oftentimes, with the freedom of campus life comes a price. Without the boundaries of parents' expectations or the structure provided by tightly-knit social groups formed in high school, AD/HD students can become overwhelmed and isolated, turning to marijuana or alcohol and/or falling into the wrong social crowd quickly.

Why is it so difficult?

In the AD/HD population, there exists a wide spectrum of social skills abilities—those who are extremely adept socially and those who aren't. In many cases, other specific brain issues or learning disabilities affect social skills, and AD/HD is only a small part of the problem. However, for the purposes of this book, the focus is *only* on how AD/HD can affect and inhibit social skill development and how a coach can help. For those who have other complicating factors, it is suggested that they seek the help of a professional who specializes in social skills training.

Despite one's social skill abilities or disabilities, the college setting holds many social challenges for students with AD/HD. College requires more self-imposed structure and can exacerbate the very symptoms of AD/HD that interfere with social interactions—impulsiveness, inattentiveness, forgetfulness, and distractibility. Students with AD/HD have to work extra hard at developing social skills. Otherwise, the effects of their AD/HD on social situations can be seen as character flaws or translate into labels such as loud, obnoxious, self-centered, inconsiderate, spacey, or nerdy. Because they had a history with peers and teachers in high school, quirky behavior might have been overlooked or accepted. In college, judgments can be made quickly; first impressions are formed faster and at times hold more weight. What was tolerated in high school, won't be in college or the workplace—the rules have changed.

How does coaching help?

Perhaps one of the most important functions of an AD/HD coach is that of "social skills monitor." Developing social skills requires the ability to read social rules and match one's conduct to those rules. To do this one must listen, pay attention, self-observe, and then self-correct and modulate one's own behavior according to the situation. Through coaching, students can learn from past experiences, identify, anticipate, and prepare for interactions or situations that are challenging or difficult. The coaching partnership provides a safe place to slow down, ask questions, practice dialogues, and receive feedback regarding social skills. Also, with more choices available to them in college, students with AD/HD are likely to get overwhelmed, act impulsively, and not use good judgment in many social situations. By talking things through with the coach, students can learn to use self-talk as a way to think through the consequences of potential actions. Coaching can help build independence by increasing one's confidence and trust in one's own ability to make good choices.

Another challenge facing many students with AD/HD entering college is the inability to advocate for themselves. This situation may be the result of any one of several misconceptions. Some students try to shed the stigma of AD/HD they felt they had in high school, and often won't ask for accommodations in college until it is too late and they are failing classes. Some of these students think college is the time to prove they can do it on their own, without special help, while other students never really learned to self-advocate because others always advocated on their behalf (parents or teachers) and they never learned what to ask for to enhance successful performance.

Working with a coach helps students to identify and acknowledge their brain differences. With the support and encouragement of a coach, students can explore strategies and methods to help them become more independent. The coaching process itself helps students develop a language to describe what they are experiencing and creates an opportunity to practice asking for what they need— an essential life skill.

College is a time of personal discovery and growth for all young adults. Making new friends and creating lifelong memories are part of campus life and of the college experience. College is a springboard—a testing ground—for all students to learn necessary life skills. For the student with AD/HD, it is imperative that this time be taken seriously. Reading and understanding cultural rules is necessary to life beyond college and impacts one's personal life and intimate relationships. Understanding more subtle social cues and being able to manage one's impulses to act appropriately can be the fine line between fitting in or being isolated.

Working with a coach can help the student to know and understand himself, the effects of his disability, and how these play in social interactions. The key to developing social skills is knowing how to apply this knowledge. The guidance of and partnership with a coach will help provide a place to learn and practice the details of intricate social skills. The process of coaching will help the student to remember the importance of social skills and be prepared for life beyond college by bridging the gap between knowing and doing. Over time, with feedback, encouragement and motivation from the coach—the student with AD/HD can develop tools to help him be successful and negotiate social situations in the future.

Issue:

Making friends

Understanding the Issue

Many factors influence making friends in college. Whether you attend a large or a small school, live on or off campus, or are a full or part-time student, all affect the ability to make friends. Especially in the beginning, before areas of concentration are declared, college provides little consistency in terms of prolonged contact with the same group of people. Changing class schedules and living situations combined with long semester breaks add to this lack of continuity. Part of what makes college unique is the constant change. Yet, one of the key factors to making friends is having regular contact over time with people who have shared interests.

Without a doubt, college can be a difficult transition from the routine high school environment. For some students with AD/HD, the novelty of college is stimulating, while for others, it is overwhelming. Regardless of one's "social abilities," a lot of conscious effort needs to go into not only making friends, but also choosing the right ones.

A coach can help a student keep his social life in check. By working with a coach, the student can create methods and ways to meet and aline himself with other students who have similar interests and goals. Most importantly, a coach can help the student plan a social life by scheduling dates with friends and reminding him that school is just as much about growing socially as it is academically!

It is important to mention, however, that while working with a coach can help the student identify how his AD/HD helps or hinders the process of making friends and develop practical strategies to make friends, coaches are not trained social skills specialists. If problems persist in the area of making friends, students with AD/HD are encouraged to seek a medical evaluation and to explore other issues that might be causing problems. Trained professionals such as a therapists, psychiatrists, speech and language therapists, or a social skills specialist can aide in this process.

Addressing the Issue

The coach can help the student:

Make AD/HD a friend. The first step in helping a student to make friends with others is aiding him in understanding his own AD/HD and examining how it affects him in social situations. Identifying strengths, as well as helping him to acknowledge challenges, is all part of accepting his brain differences.

Identify the barriers. Explore with the student what is preventing him from making friends. Is it a matter of making it a priority—of not creating time for friends? Or is it more skill based—for example, not knowing how to start a conversation? If you can identify what some of the barriers are, then you and the student can work on how to devise ways to get around them.

Take action. Work with the student to take action toward making changes. If there are things that prevent him from making friends, help him gather the courage to take corrective measures. For example, does he avoid people because he doesn't know how to maintain eye contact? Is personal grooming an issue? These things might not have been that important in the past, but they can hinder the process of making friends and may need to be worked on now. Bring these issues to the forefront of the coaching process so the two of you might work on them.

Set clear coaching goals. By establishing "making friends" as a goal, the student will be more likely to work toward this goal and thus achieve it. Encourage the student to set up clear guidelines as to what he wants to achieve (make one new friend per semester, make friends with one person in each class, etc.).

Be accountable. Encourage the student to use the coach as the much needed "environmental tool" to make sure he follows through on his plans. Often, if AD/HD students make plans, they forget about them, or have a last minute "mood" change and do something else. With continued reminders from the coach, the student can be sure to keep "making friends" a priority.

Break down the process. Break down the process into doable steps with the student. This will help the student to understand and learn the process of how to make friends. As a coach you can help the student to:

- Identify and pursue his interests. Encourage the student to join clubs or groups that interest him and attend them on a regular basis. A student is more likely to meet people more easily, if he knows others already share a common interest.

- Increase social opportunities. This is a simple rule of math that should be shared with the student: one's chances of making friends increases with the number of times one goes out. The more people they come in contact with, the more likely they are to find someone with whom they can become friends. Sitting at home watching TV will not help them meet friends. Stress the importance of going out and making the effort.

- Create time and space for making friends. Have the student work with you to set up a plan to be social. Have him block out time and space for social events. Help him plan for these events by marking them on his schedule and calendar. Many AD/HD students don't plan because they want to keep their options open and end up without tickets or seats at a concert

or movie. Making friends is not something that happens—
one must make plans and create room for it in life.

- Anticipate and rehearse encounters. Reinforce the importance
  of preparing for social encounters. Create social scripts with
  the student and have him practice them with you. This will
  help them to get beyond the initial "Hi, how are you?" and
  helps him to learn ways to ask the second question. For example, a second question might be, "What did you think of
  Prof. Jones's test?" Other scripts might include asking questions about others. This helps to demonstrate interest in them,
  but can also help the student to "stay curious" so as to sustain
  attention to conversations. Anticipating and practicing the flow
  of conversations and sequence of events helps students to make
  these skills more natural.

Understand the importance of nonverbal communication. What
the eye cannot see the mind will read. Even the most socially
adept student with AD/HD can underestimate the importance of
nonverbal social abilities. This includes reading non-verbal cues,
as well as learning what nonverbal messages he is sending. Discuss with the student strategies to help him be more present so he
can read and act on other people's needs. This means paying attention to voice intonations, facial expressions, etc. On his end,
learning to maintain eye contact (without staring), learning to act
like he is listening, and learning how to use his body appropriately (standing still, facing the person speaking to them, etc.) are
all very important skills to learn.

Use the coaching relationship. Have the student give you
permission to offer feedback on his social skills. This means
being nonjudgemental and helping the student to trust you, so he
can be open to hearing observations and receiving suggestions on
how to improve. Remember, most social skills are learned. So use
your interactions with the student as a way to teach him some of
these skills.

Issue:	
	Keeping friends

Understanding the Issue

Many students entering college have grown up in the same town, all or most of their lives. Friendships have been formed through their local communities, schools, families, or clubs (sports, arts, etc.). The bond of time can create friends who are tolerant and forgiving of the symptoms of AD/HD. This can create a false sense of security in that not much work has gone in to keeping these particular friends. Keeping friends in college is different. A conscious and continued effort of attending to the details of friendship has to be made in order to maintain friendships.

Numerous issues affect the AD/HD student's ability to keep friends. Often, students with AD/HD are perceived by others as self-centered, too intense, irresponsible, or undependable. Keeping friends is hard work. There is no way around it. It takes time, effort, and persistence. A coach can help the student remember this priority and work with him to devise ways to pay attention and attend to the details of maintaining friendships.

Addressing the Issue

The coach can help the student:

Know himself. Your job as coach is to foster the student's knowledge of his AD/HD tendencies. This is key to the process of developing self-understanding. For example, if the student knows he or she forgets appointments, can't remember names, doesn't return calls, can't commit to weekend plans, talks too much, or gets bored easily, remind him or her of these things. Help the student acknowledge these tendencies and the negative results they can cause.

Together, you and the student can create ways to improve performance in these areas.

Be vigilant. Making good friends takes time. Once a friend is made, it is easy to get lazy. AD/HD students are famous for starting out very intense in relationships. This can form a strong bond in some cases, but often not enough to sustain the friendship over time. In order to keep friends, one needs to work at it, making himself available to the relationship, keeping commitments, and staying in touch on a regular basis. This means taking responsibility to do what is necessary to keep and maintain friendships.

Get organized. Help the student understand the value of organization to keeping friends. Is losing telephone numbers and addresses a major issue? Or forgetting birthdays or other important dates? Work with the student to mark these important dates on a calendar or in an address and phone list. Simple organizational techniques can save time and help keep friends.

Create rituals and routines. Stress the importance of planning regular activities with friends. Have the student center meetings around the same activity—a weekly tennis game, coffee at 8 AM on Fridays, a weekly jog, etc. These rituals are extremely valuable in helping to create lasting friendships. Help the student to set aside the time, to be accountable to you for keeping these appointments, and to not let anything get in the way.

Think small and get big results. The small things in friendship count—remembering a friend's birthday, showing support by attending games or performances, calling just to say "hi," emailing a get well card, etc. These may seem like unimportant details, but make a big impact on keeping friends and show you really care. Have the student designate a calendar for birthdays and post it so he can see it all the time. Have him share the dates with you and other details about their friends (e.g. "Sam has a game Friday"). These dates should be marked on his weekly schedule, just as he would mark an exam date. Make the student accountable to you for following through on these commitments.

Make intentions a reality. Most AD/HD students have great intentions—they *intend* to make plans, to call this person or that person, they *intend* to make a lunch date, go to a movie, or play a game of basketball—but never do it. Work with the student on getting these ideas out of his head and making them a reality. By talking with the coach, a student can make these intentions more concrete (i.e. meet at least one friend for lunch every week, etc.) Create accountability around these intentions, so they can be turned into actions.

Know the limits of using intuition. Many AD/HD students are extremely intuitive and make friends easily because of their ability to understand and read other people. However, this same ability can be a liability. If there is an overreliance on intuition, it can make the student lazy and feel that he doesn't need to pay attention to the other person. Most persons with AD/HD will claim they know what the person is going to say before they say it, so they don't need to listen. This attitude can get them into trouble by assuming too much. Friendships are two-way streets. Stress the importance of keeping engaged, asking for feedback, and not to ever assume what someone else is thinking without verification. A coach can help the student to practice slowing down and mirror back what is heard from the conversation. The coaching relationship can provide a safe place to practice these types of skills and receive feedback without fear of losing a friend.

Set boundaries. Because of their sensitivity and intuitiveness many students with AD/HD become "counselors" to others. Their willingness to be generous with their time and not to think of the consequences can take its toll on their lives. Some students report missing classes, delaying studying, and failing an exam because they were taking better care of others needs than they did their own. Coaches can help students become aware of these patterns and learn ways to set boundaries while still being caring.

Be aware that problems in friendship could signal a problem. The coach can help the student look at these issues and decide if problems with friendships are signaling the need for a referral to a therapist or counselor for more help in unraveling the emotional issues contributing to the difficulties.

Issue:

Getting along with roommates

Understanding the Issue

At an AD/HD conference, a parent was overheard to say, "After seeing the disaster in my son's room, only a mother could love him!" Oftentimes, parents do a disservice to their children by not teaching and requiring them to follow through on personal responsibilities, such as keeping their rooms clean or picking up after themselves. In college, dirty laundry piled all over the room can make enemies of roommates or friends. Whether the student shares a dorm room or an apartment, the small details count. When it comes to sharing space or living with others, not changing the toilet paper, leaving messes, not washing the dishes, or buying groceries carries a lot of weight.

In the past, perhaps other people reminded the student to pick up his messes or did it for him. Although it is not intentional, this lack of personal responsibility can affect all relationships—from intimate to professional.

It is worth mentioning here that it is not always the student with AD/HD that is the disorganized or messy one. Often, students with AD/HD need to have their environment neat and chaos-free, almost as a way to balance their disorganized minds. This might mean an environment that has minimal distractions and few noise disturbances. This poses special challenges as quiet living places are rarely found in most campus living situations.

College can be the first time that some students with AD/HD must learn to live in a group outside of their own families, while others might have gone to private schools or camps and are familiar with group living. Regardless of one's prior group living experiences, effectively communicating your needs, being able to maintain your personal space, reading and respecting other people's needs, and knowing how to be a "team player," is important.

Addressing the Issue

The coach can help the student:

Identify needs. Being up front about one's AD/HD and how it affects daily living is an important skill for students to develop. Coaches can help students to verbalize and explain the symptoms they might display (being forgetful, not paying attention to details, and getting overwhelmed with lots of noise) are not deliberate or intentional acts, rather are part of their AD/HD. Encourage students to be honest and direct and discuss ways to deal with these issues before they cause a problem. Coaches can work with students to offer suggestions on how people can help them if they are falling short of their responsibilities. Stress the importance of having them ask how it is best to approach others if their needs are not being met. So, whether the student is the messy type that needs reminders to pick up after him or herself, or if he requires a neat environment, learning to communicate this message is key. Rehearsing and practicing with a coach can help to expedite this process.

Identify areas of challenges. Many AD/HD students have a pretty good idea of what areas they need to improve—mostly because they have been nagged or teased about their living habits by parents, siblings, and friends. Coaches can role play with students to help them learn to be up front with new roommates by saying, "I am known for being messy, but I'm used to being nagged about it, so don't be afraid to say something if my messes get too bad!" This brings the issue immediately into the open and can help reduce concerns others may have about what to say to them once they experience their messes.

Create a personal checklist. Have students create a checklist of duties they need to do on a regular basis to maintain their personal space. This might include a sequence of activities they would follow each day (wake up, pick up clothes, wash breakfast dishes, clean up bathroom, clear study space, etc.). Suggest they post this checklist and check it off each day until it becomes habit. Reinforce using the checklist by having them be accountable to you for filling it out. This will help them remain vigilant in the areas in which they are weak. Over time, they will internalize some of these basic living skills. The time spent on this now will be well worth it. By doing this, the student will then have established habits that will remain with him for future living situations.

Keep lines of communication open. Frequently, AD/HD students wait for someone to complain about something they have done, before asking for feedback. Urge the student to take the initiative to communicate about these issues in a direct manner. By doing this, it will help him to make others feel more comfortable in expressing their feelings—both positive and negative—about his living habits.

Keep things nontoxic. Encourage the student to brainstorm with his living partners ways to communicate effectively as a group and with one another. Suggest that ground rules be set for what is and is not acceptable. Stress the importance of removing emotions. Getting angry, blaming, or taking things personally will only escalate bad situations and create more tension. Having weekly meetings or posting a chore list on a message board are examples of ways to not let things build up among the group.

Make it a group effort. Help students avoid becoming a scapegoat. If they know they tend to lose keys, forget to pay bills, and lose phone messages have them set up ways for these details to become a group responsibility. Have them find out what other people have difficulties with and make it a group mission to brainstorm ideas on how, as a group, they can help each other. Here are simple ways other AD/HD students have handled some of these situations: posting a message board by the phone; marking bill due-dates on a group calendar and reminding each other of the dates; have one person who is good with details handle the bills; make extra copies of apartment keys; post a colorful note by the sink saying, "Remember to wash your own dishes."

Issue:

Getting along in group situations

Understanding the Issue

College is filled with numerous types of group interactions ranging from class discussions, study groups, group projects, to receptions and parties.

Some AD/HD students mature more slowly than their peers. This delay in development can show up as a lack of social skills. Social skills are weighed more heavily in group situations. Simple things like laughing when a joke is told, waiting one's turn to talk, not interrupting others, following and adding to conversations, and responding to comments appropriately, are all part of having well-developed social skills.

When it comes to group projects, it is important for students to understand what their responsibilities are to the group and to follow through on them. It is not only the student's grade that will be affected by not contributing, but also the grades of all group members.

Addressing the Issue

The coach can help the student:

Identify challenges and create strategies. By having the student work through the details of his difficulties, problem areas can more easily be isolated. Together the student and the coach can create strategies to help successfully manage group situations. Below are some strategies that many AD/HD students have found useful:

Strategies for study groups or group projects

- Have the student view study groups as his friend. Some of the best learning happens in small discussion groups. This is particularly true for students with AD/HD. The conversations are more intense and targeted. Stress that he should never miss an opportunity to attend these groups.

- Have him review the purpose and agenda of the group before each meeting (either from his notes or with a group participant). This helps to keep the big picture in mind and better focus attention on the discussion.

- Encourage openness about AD/HD. Encourage the student to share with the group any difficulties he might experience in group settings, so he can get the assistance he needs (reminders, feedback, etc.). However, AD/HD should not be used as an excuse for falling short of obligations or acting inappropriately.

- Suggest that the student partner with someone in the group to review major points after each group meeting. This way he can make sure he is catching all the main points along with reinforcing the learning process.

- Suggest using a tape recorder to tape group sessions. (To save time, some students note the number on the tape gauge during parts of the discussion they don't understand. This way they can review only these parts and not have to listen to the entire tape.)

- Have the student ask to get a copy of someone else's notes from the group, if he has a hard time taking notes.

- Suggest that all instructions be obtained in writing. This way the student can post them and refer back to them when needed.

- Work with the student to mark all deadlines and responsibilities for the group project on a calendar. Have him post it where it will be seen often so he doesn't fall short of his duties to the group.

- Remind the student to not overcommit. It is easy for students with AD/HD to get carried away by the moment and to volunteer for more than they can do. Urge him to take on less than he thinks he can do. It usually turns out to be more than he thought it would be. He can also be helped to think before committing by saying, "Let me think about this."

- Have the student share all obligations, responsibilities, and due dates for work owed the group. This will create the extra accountability needed to make sure he follows through.

Strategies for social group situations

- Help the student understand the type of event he is attending and related details before arriving. Have him be sure to ask advice from the host or a friend about proper dress, time of arrival, and if he is expected to contribute something (food, money, etc.).

- Encourage the student to observe how the pros do it. Suggest he "shadow" friends who has good social skills at a party or other social gathering. Observe how they maneuver their way in and out of conversations, how they hold their body, the distance they stand from others, etc. This can be used as a model in helping students learn group social skills.

- If small talk is hard for a student, have him prepare and rehearse questions to ask others. This can help in initiating conversations.

- If a student tends to talk too much, have him prepare a list of questions to ask others. This can help in learning the skill of showing interest in others, as well as helping him to not talk as much.

- Encourage the student to ask a good friend to give him an honest assessment of how he handles himself in group situations. Have him ask for feedback and specific suggestions on how to improve himself in this area. Does he maintain enough eye contact? Does he talk too loudly? Too softly? Does he stand too close?

- Practice, practice, practice! In order to gain group social skills, the student must attend group functions and practice. Encourage him to make this one of his coaching goals and to attend several functions per semester.

- If a student tends to "space out" at group events or get bored, be sure to stress that he not sit down. Have him stand or walk around. This helps to activate the brain and will allow him to maintain his attention better.

- If a student tends to get overwhelmed in groups, help him to try to keep his focus. Have him move away from noisy areas and pick one or two persons with whom to talk.

- Set specific goals with the student and create accountability to follow through on them. For example, have him initiate conversations with two people at a group function, listen more, talk less, not interrupt as much, etc.

Issue:

**Establishing balance
in romantic relationships**

Understanding the Issue

No matter if a person has AD/HD or not, college is a time of experimentation, self-exploration and discovery of personal limits. Falling in love for the first time and spending countless hours with a romantic partner is a natural occurrence and happens to many college students. However, AD/HD students can be "all or nothing" in the area of romance, and it is the extremes that can become worrisome. One extreme is the AD/HD student who falls in love deeply and often—who lets intimate relationships become all-consuming to the point where academic goals get lost. The other extreme is the student who never dates and lives in perpetual loneliness due to his or her inability to foster intimate relationships.

In high school, parents are present to monitor these situations and set limits, or push and prod a little. This is not so in college. Students are expected to achieve balance in their lives on their own— an ability that is hard for many students with AD/HD to learn. Understanding the importance of striking a balance between romance and academics oftentimes does not occur until after severe consequences have resulted from one extreme or the other.

A coach can help students with AD/HD with this delicate balancing act by helping keep identified goals in mind. By doing this, students are then able to set up preventive measures and strategies so as not to veer too far to one extreme or the other.

Addressing the Issue

The coach can help the student:

Make balance a coaching goal. This requires the student to first know how he gets "out of balance." For example, if he knows the moves toward extremes when it comes to dating and striking a balance is hard, have him program you to remind him of this fact. This is the perfect time for him to work on this all-or-nothing life style. Here are coaching strategies for both cases:

> ## Loving and *not learning*:
> ## Spending too much time in love.

- **Create "red flags" with the coach.** Encourage the student to explore where his danger zones lie. If he is the type of person who loses himself or gets "taken by the moment" when it comes to romance, red flag the situations in which this occurs. For instance, if a student knows that staying the night with his date will lead to him spending days or weeks together, get permission to remind the student of this. He can then develop ways to prevent the cycle before it starts.

- **Have reality checks with the coach.** One of the hazards of AD/HD is not measuring time well. What feels like a couple of hours spent with one's partner each day can in reality be a lot more. Suggest that the student keep a log of how much time he spends with his significant other and share it with the coach. Oftentimes, this can be eye opening and help a student redirect himself to his studies.

- **Get help from the partner.** Encourage the student to use you to help him come up with ways to explain his impulsive tendencies to potential romantic partners. And especially how this leads to his losing site of his academic goals. Have him practice asking for help from his partner in keeping to his study schedules and in being practical about how much time they are spending together.

- **Be accountable to the coach.** Encourage the student to use the coach to help him set limits for himself. Have him check-in regularly on his progress in upholding these boundaries. Without accountability to the coach, chances are he will not have the much-needed willpower to stay the course.

> ### Learning and *not loving:*
> ### Spending too much time studying.

- **Identify what gets in the way.** If all a student does is study and never dates, encourage him or her to identify what is getting in the way. Is it an issue of time management? Is he spending weekends in the library catching up on studies? Or is it something else? Create the space for him to be honest and open. By talking things through, the coach can help him to confront these barriers and develop strategies to maneuver around them.

- **Make dating a coaching goal.** If a student knows that he tends to avoid asking people out on dates, have him make it a goal and develop a plan on how he will go about making dating a reality in college. Set up measurable steps so he can see progress. For example, attend three social events, join a social club, and ask one new person out every month, etc.

- **Create accountability with the coach.** Have the student be accountable for following through on dating plans. Without accountability, plans are less likely to become a reality.

ACADEMIC SKILLS— ISSUES FOR COLLEGE STUDENTS WITH AD/HD

What is it all about?

Although college students with AD/HD may have intellectual abilities and academic skills that surpass those of their non-disabled peers, they are at greater risk for not succeeding at college. The success that many students with AD/HD experienced in the structured, supervised world of high school may not continue when they go off to college. All students face a host of academic and non-academic decisions as they enter college. This transition requires adjustments to many new experiences and expectations. Performance problems exhibited by students with AD/HD, coupled with the higher thinking skill deficiencies caused by their disability can cause a host of issues as they transition to the unstructured, unsupervised world of college. College students with AD/HD encounter a range of problems and decisions as they attempt to select a schedule, learn to listen in large lecture classes, form new study habits and routines, and begin to manage the complex, long-term assignments they are given.

How does coaching help?

Current research and growing clinical experience has shown that accommodations alone are not enough to allow students with AD/HD to succeed academically. The unique partnership of a coaching relationship can provide the external structure, support, and accountability college students with AD/HD need to help them achieve to their full potential. A coach can be a trusted partner, helping the student learn to develop routines, habits, and skills needed to handle the academic tasks and decisions they encounter at college. By allowing the student to drive the process as he learns to handle the challenges he encounters, coaching can foster opportunities for academic and personal growth. Coaching is designed to help students remind themselves of their overall goals, as well as the steps they need to take to reach these goals. Coaching not only assists students in setting up programs to get their work done, but also helps them observe and regulate their own behaviors in the process. By working with a coach, students develop the kind of self-awareness needed to identify and work from their strengths, and to replace weak or ineffective skills and habits with more effective ones.

Issue:

Scheduling classes

Understanding the Issue

Selecting a class schedule is one of the first major decisions college students make. While they may have had some choice over the specific subjects that took in high school, there is a great deal of freedom in what courses to take and when to take them during any given semester in college. There are catalogs, online sites about classes, advisors, and other resource people available to help students make these decisions. However, whether students choose to consult these resources and how helpful such supports may be will vary greatly. Many students opt to rely on the informal advising network made up of older siblings or friends who attended college, or the information available behind the scenes in fraternities, sororities, and other student organizations.

Consequently, it is not unusual for freshmen to make questionable decisions about their first semester's schedule. They may naively select classes based on limited criteria and not think through all the factors to consider, including: class size, work required, how the class fits with other classes taken that semester, information about the professors teaching style, etc. Students also have to learn to pay careful attention to the deadlines for adding and dropping courses so changes can be made in a particularly challenging schedule before it is too late. It can also be overwhelming for freshman to adjust to the process of registration on most campuses. Deadlines are established for when the registration system is open for each group of students (graduates, seniors, juniors, sophomores, and freshmen). At the preordained time, students must persist at calling a computerized system or going online to get their schedules. Most learn quickly that they have to have plans A, B, and C ready since they rarely get their first choice of courses. Learning from experience, students typically become adept at making better selections to ensure that their schedules are more balanced.

The AD/HD brain can also make the process of selecting a class schedule quite difficult. Registering for classes depends on a host of skills that are not easy for the individual with AD/HD. Given their tendency toward impulsive thinking, it is likely that college students with AD/HD will have difficulty reflecting on all the important factors in selecting a class schedule that is a good match to his or her needs. Furthermore, it can be extremely challenging for the student with AD/HD to stay on top of the paperwork and the deadlines for registration. Learning to use a computerized registration system can be a barrier for some students who have trouble following the complex directions for this process. Difficulties in problem-solving can make registration time quite stressful as college students with AD/HD try to register and discover that their initial plan won't work. They may have difficulty seeing an alternative plan and react emotionally when their first choices for classes aren't available. Unlike their nondisabled peers, students with AD/HD may not productively analyze the problems they've experienced and learn from previous mistakes. Instead, they may repeat the same pattern each semester, postponing dealing with registration until the last minute, selecting an unbalanced schedule or one that is not matched to their needs. It is not uncommon for college students with AD/HD to continue to schedule early morning classes in hopes that this will force them into a daily structure, or to simply forget about spacing out their classes to allow time to take medication, breaks, or to eat lunch.

A relationship with a coach can increase the likelihood that college students with AD/HD will think more about the schedules they select and meet the deadlines in the registration process. By agreeing to be coached on selecting a schedule, students with AD/HD can be helped to plan ahead and follow the plan that is created. The coach can help the student actually take all the steps necessary to select a schedule rather than forget about this process until the last minute.

By posing the right questions, the coach can encourage the student to learn from past experience and think more critically about a potential schedule. With the help of a coach, the college student with AD/HD can identify questions and concerns about courses and talk with the appropriate resource people available on campus. College students with AD/HD may be eligible for early registration, which is a legally mandated accommodation on most campuses. The coach can encourage the student to seek out the disabilities services office to determine if he or she qualifies. Early registration allows students with disabilities to register before all other students and can increase the likelihood that a balanced schedule is selected. Even if the student does qualify, he or she will need to think through a schedule and have all paperwork in order by a specified date.

Addressing the Issue

The coach can help the student:

1 Develop internal structures by learning from past experience.

Examples:

- Make a list of tips for selecting a balanced schedule based on the student's past experience.

- Interview other people (advisors, older students, relatives, and friends) and add their tips to the list.

- Sample tips may include:

  - Always register for an extra class so there's one to drop if one class is not a good match.

  - Leave room between classes so you can get from class

to class without rushing and so there is time to take medication or get a snack.

- Take tough classes when you are most alert and easier classes when you are least alert.

- Take the fewest hours possible until you are better adjusted to college.

- Choose a balance of courses that are required and electives that you like.

- Consider taking the smaller sections of classes even if the time of day isn't perfect.

2 Plan ahead.

Examples:

- Make a checklist of all the small steps in selecting a class schedule.

- Meet with advisor to see what courses are needed.

- Get information about course requirements.

- Rate difficulty level of each class.

- Identify the best times for classes and breaks and make a master schedule by copying the time schedule that is usually available in registration materials.

- Go online and identify several course sections for each class.

- Make up several possible schedules.

3 Set very specific goals for daily action.

Example:

- Use the checklist to identify small actions to take each day, like call advisor to schedule a meeting or go online for 10 minutes to look at possible courses.

◼4 Develop external structures.

Examples:
- Be accountable to the coach for taking each action on the checklist. Call or email when the step is complete.

- Program the coach or a friend to give helpful reminders to get things done.

- Organize all registration materials into a notebook to be used each semester. Have the coach keep copies of everything, just in case.

◼5 Engineer the environment.

Examples:
- Make a list of all the benefits of getting registration done early and post these in a visible place.

- Develop a self-reward system for taking each small step on the checklist.

- Work with a buddy and make selecting a schedule fun. Set a lunch date at a nice restaurant to talk over course selections.

- Use coaching meetings to actually do the tedious steps that are being put off, like reading the course catalogs or going online to collect information.

◼6 Monitor progress.

Examples:
- Use the master checklist to record dates when tasks are completed. Do this at the start of each coaching meeting.

- Lay out target dates for completion of each step on a monthly calendar and review at each coaching meeting.

Issue:

**Paying attention
and taking notes**

Understanding the Issue

The transition to college requires adjustments to many new experiences and expectations. New students often experience some stress during the adjustment period when they discover that learning goes on in large lecture classes with little or no student interaction. Unlike high school, college courses typically consist of large lecture classes (from 50 to several hundred students) in which class meetings are used to impart the course information. In fact, at some large universities the lectures are actually videotaped and students sit in large auditoriums watching a video of a previously recorded lecture. Although textbooks and other reading assignments may be the foundation for the course, the lecture itself is where the professor ties together readings with important information from his or her own research and study. While some discussion or active learning may go on during small group recitation classes, for many basic courses like (Biology, History, Sociology, etc.) the student is expected to just listen and learn in a lecture. A class period may last for fifty minutes or as long as several hours.

To survive in this type of learning environment, new freshmen have to quickly refine their note-taking skills, which were probably underused during high school. Given good attention, good self-control, and well-developed problem-solving skills, most freshmen are capable of generating new tools to listen, sit still, and take notes in their classes. When trouble arises, they probably have no difficulty asking the professor or their friends for help to fill in any gaps that might exist in their notes. They most likely seek out note-taking resources like study skill books, workshops, and note-taking services available on most campuses or on the Internet.

It is quite obvious why a college student with AD/HD may have serious problems remaining attentive and alert during a lecture and difficulty taking class notes. For many students with this disability, being in a passive learning situation is, by far, their greatest challenge. As long as they are moving or interacting with information in some way, they are usually more capable of remaining awake, alert, and focused. The range of problems a student with AD/HD has while listening and taking notes may vary depending on a number of factors, including the subject matter and how interesting it is to the student, where the student sits, the lecturer's style of teaching, the use of audio-visual materials to supplement the lecture, the time of day, the number of hours the student has been in class already, the student's skill at being an active listener, and how effective the student's medication is at the time of the lecture.

While some students with AD/HD have excellent verbal abilities and prefer listening as a way to learn, others report having tremendous difficulty keeping their minds focused on spoken information. For some students, the problem is very basic. They are unable to remain awake and alert in such a setting. Others may struggle to simply sit still for the duration of the class without the opportunity to get up and stretch. Some students with distractible minds complain that ideas shared in a lecture trigger a stream of consciousness that leads them to lose track of what the professor is saying. By the time they catch themselves from drifting with an idea, they have already lost important information that was spoken but not written anywhere. Others describe feeling very stressed as they work frantically to record what was said without being able to actually understand the information being taught. In the rush to record their notes, many students with AD/HD express frustration because they have illegible, disorganized, and incomplete class notes that cannot be used to review and study the lecture. The negative feelings created by their difficulties in lecture settings can lead some students to begin avoiding these classes altogether, placing them at great risk for failure or very poor grades.

By forming a relationship with a coach, a college student with AD/HD can identify and implement productive ways to overcome the problem of listening during a lecture and taking notes. The coaching partnership can allow the student to openly discuss the stresses and challenges they experience in lecture classes and to develop very personalized methods for dealing with these difficulties. An important function of a coach is to encourage students with AD/HD to uncover campus resources for improving note-taking skills, or for receiving accommodations for this problem from a campus disability service provider. The coaching relationship can also be a safe place for the student to practice talking about his or her disability and learning how to advocate for help with professors. By being accountable to a coach, students can be helped to follow through on their plans and work toward preventing these problems from turning into much larger academic issues.

Addressing the Issue

The coach can help the student:

1 **Engineer the environment to make paying attention easier.**

Examples:

- Pick a seat that makes focusing and paying attention possible. Seats in the front of the class may be the best for tuning out distractions, however, they are not the best if the student needs a stretch break midway through class. Getting a prime seat requires getting to class early.

- Time medication and meals to be matched to lecture

classes to increase the ability to remain awake, alert, and focused.

- When registering for a semester, balance the day with lecture classes, breaks, and movement classes.

- If allowed, have food, candy, gum, or water available to help with remaining alert.

- Get permission from the professor to tape the lectures using a tape player with a counter. Whenever the student's attention drifts, mark the counter number in the margin of the paper and replay that section of the tape.

- Talk to the professor and discuss how AD/HD is impacting listening and note-taking. (While this is a difficult task for many students who may not be comfortable disclosing their disability and needs with the professor, it has the potential to elicit productive solutions to the problem. Once a professor knows what type of problem a student is having, they frequently offer help and support that solves the problem. It is not unusual for professors to offer students a copy of their overhead transparencies or Powerpoint slides to make note-taking easier. Some professors have also offered an actual copy of their notes. If students need to get up and stretch during the lecture, the professor may be willing to give a short break to the entire class to stand up and stretch during long lectures. On several occasions, professors have offered to meet with students after class to help them fill in gaps in their class notes.)

2 **Set very specific goals for note taking during coaching sessions.**

Examples:
- Define how the student will head the page for taking notes: date, course, topic.

- Set the goal of reviewing the previous day's notes before class to get ready for listening.

- Set a goal for how many pages of notes the student will try to take.

- Commit to spending time right after class reviewing notes and filling in gaps by talking with other students or the professor.

3 Develop internal structures.

Examples:

- Learn how to take notes by attending a workshop or meeting with a college disability services provider.

- Wear a watch that beeps and use this as a reminder to ask, "Was I paying attention?" or some other phrase that promotes self-monitoring.

- Ask a friend to sit nearby and provide a signal if he or she notices the student "drifting."

4 Observe what contributes to the note-taking problems.

Examples:

- Send an email to the coach after each class rating how note-taking went and list what helped and what got in the way.

- Read the student's psychoeducational evaluation together and make a list of what factors contribute to problems taking notes. Make a plan to deal with each factor.

5 Develop external structures that promote taking notes.

Examples:

- Be accountable to the coach on a daily basis for taking notes. Send email, voice mail, or other messages reporting on progress taking notes.

- Design a personalized reward system for taking notes.

Issue:

Managing long-term
assignments

Understanding the Issue

Learning how to complete a host of complex assignments that are not due for a long period of time is one of the most challenging expectations usually encountered during the transition to college. It is not uncommon for college classes to have only two exams: a mid-term and a final. Such classes require the student to stay current on the voluminous reading assignments listed on a syllabus. In some classes, several very complex writing assignments may be used to evaluate the student's knowledge of reading assignments that are never even discussed in class. In other instances, professors may assign one large research paper or a project that is due on the last day of class. In all instances, there may be little or no discussion in class of how to structure progress on these types of assignments, as well as little or no reminding about the actual due date.

This is in stark contrast to what students typically experienced in high school, where daily homework is assigned, collected, and graded. To ensure that students are making progress on hefty reading assignments, teachers may have pop quizzes or ask the student to keep a journal of his or her reactions to the readings. Tests tend to occur frequently on a weekly or bi-weekly basis. When teachers assign research papers to prepare students for college, many tend to break the task up into several stages and assign due dates for collecting portions of the work. For example, a student may need to hand in a paragraph describing the topic selected for a history research paper during one week, an annotated bibliography of the sources cited during another, an outline of the paper may need to be handed in and approved, and so on. Finally, the teacher may collect a draft of the paper that is circulated among class members for feedback several weeks before collecting the final copy. Even when high school teachers don't structure long-term assignments this carefully, they are likely to provide reminders about the due dates in class. For the most part, few freshmen come from a high school setting that prepares them for the reality they will face in college with long-term assignments.

It isn't uncommon for entering freshmen to flounder initially as they adjust to this situation. They may get a low grade on their first mid-term exam and learn quickly that they need to break up the reading assignments for the next part of the semester. Some students will learn their lesson after pulling too many all nighters, trying to write a 20-page research paper or cramming for a final. In fact, many college students learn to break big tasks up into smaller, more manageable chunks through this trial-and-error approach to learning. They may turn to friends and older, more respected siblings or fraternity or sorority members to get advice on how to do a better job of managing long-term assignments during the second semester of their freshman year.

To be successful at managing long-term assignments, a college student must have a number of skills. First, it is imperative to have a keen awareness of time, the ability to analyze complex tasks into their component parts, the ability to lay out a sequential plan that can reasonably be accomplished in time, and then the ability to manage the actual implementation of that plan. College students with AD/HD are likely to have *serious difficulty* with these important planning processes. Various experts in the field of AD/HD have pointed out that individuals with this disorder tend to live in the here and now and have limitations planning in advance for events with distant due dates. The urgent tasks of today get onto their priority lists, which tends to be generated without a careful analysis of what events and tasks are hiding out of sight in the future. Consequently, many individuals with AD/HD seem to be in a chronic state of deadline-driven, intense action. To the non-AD/HD onlooker, it appears that this stressful pattern could totally be avoided if *"they had just planned ahead."* But, using their thoughts in this manner is exactly what individuals with AD/HD have difficulty doing. Most students report punishing themselves with negative messages like, "If I could just learn to plan ahead I could avoid this mess, but I never do." One gifted young woman with AD/HD offers some insight into this situation. "Unless a class is designed with frequent quizzes or graded assignments, I have no incentive or motivation to do work that isn't due until a future date. Even though I don't like the way it feels to work under the stress of a deadline, I don't see it as a consequence of my actions. Instead, to me, that deadline finally gives me the incentive and motivation I need to focus and produce. When I've tried to artificially force myself to work on a project or paper several weeks before the due date, I simply can't produce or focus. It is *so* frustrating! People might think I choose to live like this or maybe even like it. I hate it, but I can't seem to change it."

As this student's comments indicate, the cognitive consequences of AD/HD can hamper the individual's ability to break this nonproductive cycle, even when they are very motivated to do so. The natural tendencies many individuals with AD/HD have toward thinking divergently and reacting spontaneously can inhibit their ability to think of just one aspect of a task or think in a sequential fashion. As one college student with AD/HD complained, "I just can't see the small parts. I see the whole and get overwhelmed. If I have 30 articles to read in a course pack and they are all printed in a small font, I immediately react by saying, 'I'll never be able to read all these.' I get so frustrated that I don't automatically think about how I can do one article at a time." At times, students report that other issues sabotage their attempts to stop procrastinating. They may start working on a paper in advance and get stuck trying to pick a topic because they have dozens of ideas and can't choose among them. Others report logging in inordinate amounts of time in advance of a due date on a project or assignment, only to discover that they have veered off course and are working on the wrong assignment or on an interesting but nonrelated task. Others are not grounded in time and don't know what day it is, so they may think they still have plenty of time to deal with the task. Still other students report being unable to achieve the basic task of keeping track of all of their course syllabi, losing them or being unable to find them. Even if a student holds onto the syllabi, he or she may not take the time to read them periodically to see when assignments or tests are scheduled. To complicate matters, some college students with AD/HD have so many strengths that they can still get a good grade on a paper, project, or test, even when they were working like crazy to get it done at the last hour. Some students assert that they actually thrive on the rush created when they are living on the edge, trying to complete a task before the final hour. "That's when I am at my best! I am totally in hyperfocus doing my best thinking," one young man comments.

The role the coach plays in helping the student conquer long-term assignments is closely linked with the role played in the development of general planning and prioritizing skills. Many of the ideas about planning and prioritizing apply to this issue as well. However, the specific task of completing a long-term assignment deserves to be addressed separately because it come up frequently during coaching sessions and can cause so much difficulty for college students with AD/HD.

If a student is willing to work with a coach, the coaching relationship can be a vital tool in helping him or her develop new, more productive habits for dealing with long-term assignments. However, the student must be at a point where he or she has decided (not his or her parents, girlfriend, boyfriend, or frustrated roommate) that the pattern of procrastinating needs to stop. By agreeing to work with a coach to deal with this specific academic issue, a college student with AD/HD can be helped to generate systems and strategies that are more likely to work and to be used. The coaching philosophy that the student is the expert and knows what would work can remove the student's resistance toward changing old habits. By allowing the coach to function as a partner in thinking, the student may feel more hopeful that a well-developed plan will be created, remembered and actually implemented. The student may want the coach to remind him about looking at the due dates for assignments as part of his weekly contact. The student can generate the small steps for completing the task and begin working. Some students may want to think of the big picture and complete a more traditional long-term plan with tasks and due date. If the student desires, he or she can also create ways to be accountable to the coach or other individuals for taking the small steps toward completing a complex task. Some students may be helped by having to show the coach a copy of completed work as way to force action. As with planning and prioritizing, dealing more productively with the issue of long-term assignments is an essential role that coaches can play for college students with AD/HD.

Addressing the Issue

The coach can help the student:

1 Focus on the issue of dealing with long-term assignments.

In traditional approaches to teaching time management, making a semester calendar with all-important due dates is typically the first thing done when working with students. In coaching, the student drives the process, so it would be critical for the coach and student to explicitly determine if the student wants to work on this issue.

2 **Determine how the students prefers to work on long-term assignments.**

For students who agree to work on this issue, establishing the procedures for how the student wants things to be done is the first step. Some possibilities are:

- The student may, indeed, choose to create a master semester calendar that is reviewed at the start of each week or each coaching meeting. Ask the student how far ahead he or she wants to look, rather than directing this decision. Many students clearly state that they can't handle looking ahead too far in advance because they become overwhelmed seeing all the assignments that are due for several weeks, an entire month, or an entire semester.

- The student may not want to make a master calendar for the entire semester and prefer to develop a big picture calendar or task list for a smaller period of time—two weeks, three weeks, or a month.

- The student may not find having a master calendar helpful or necessary. He or she may choose, instead, to focus only on one long-term assignment with the coach rather than on broad big picture planning.

- The coach needs to ask the student in advance what role he or she wants the coach to play in reminding him or her about these tasks. Similarly, the coach needs to find out what type of feedback the student prefers when the plan is implemented and when it isn't.

3 **Promote self-observation and self-awareness.**

Examples:
- Ask the student how he or she has handled completing long-term assignments in the past. Analyze what has worked and what hasn't.

- As the student learns new ways to work on long-term assignments, keep reflecting on what helps and what hinders progress.

4 Pose questions to help analyze a task into the component parts and to select target dates for their completion.

Examples:

- Ask the student to think about what steps are involved in completing the long-term assignment or how to break the complex task into smaller manageable parts. While coaches frequently provide suggestions, the student must select an approach that he or she finds helpful so it is more likely to be used.

Examples of how students have done this are:

- Divide the pages in a large reading assignment by the number of days to complete the task and set a daily goal for reading. If the student misses a day's reading, it will need to be accounted for at another time.

- Set a daily or weekly goal for a specific amount of time to work on a long-term assignment and work with the coach to define the next small step in completion of the task. Many college students with AD/HD prefer this approach to working backward from a deadline.

- Make a specific checklist of all the steps in completing a task, like preparing for a midterm, and assign target dates for completion on a calendar. Some students, however, would rather work directly from the checklist and not assign the tasks to specific days or times.

5 **Be accountable to the coach for progress toward completion of the long-term assignment.**

Examples:

- Review progress at the start of each coaching interaction.

- The student may prefer to actually show concrete evidence of progress rather than rely on self-report. This could involve showing the work itself or telling a brief summary of what was read.

- The student may prefer to use voice mail and/or email to report on progress toward completion of a task.

6 **Be accountable to other people in the environment for progress toward completion of the long-term assignment.**

Examples:

- Encourage the student to talk openly with the professor about his need for structure in completing long-term assignments. Determine if the professor would be willing to meet periodically so the student could show progress on a paper or a project (discussing topics, research, evaluating a draft or a specific section of a paper).

- Use resource people on campus to provide the accountability the student needs to complete the small steps of a task (e.g. writing center tutors, disability service providers, counselors, or even private tutors).

- Have a friend be the student's coach and report on progress to this individual. Tell the friend in advance how and when to ask about progress and what to say if the action has or hasn't been taken.

7 Develop external structures by using rewards to motivate taking action by the target date.

Encourage the student to design a self-reward system for taking the small steps to make progress on a task. *Some examples are:*

- One student gave herself money from a savings account to purchase something special.

- Going out with friends or having a massage or some other special experience after completing a small task.

8 Develop external structures by selecting meaningful consequences for not taking action by a target date.

Examples:
Encourage the student to select consequences that he or she could institute if action isn't taken, like:

- Not going out with friends until the task is completed.

- Withholding access to TV, computer, or other rewarding activities until the task is completed.

- Giving all pleasure reading materials to a friend to hide until the task is completed.

9 Develop the internal structures/thought processes that promote taking action on the small steps toward completion of a long-term assignment.

Examples:
Have the student identify positive, meaningful messages or personal mantras or questions that might encourage taking action. Some examples students have designed and used are:

- The NIKE slogan of "JUST DO IT!"

- "You will feel so much better if you do this step now!"
- "Even though you hate doing research, it has to be done before you can write the paper."
- "Ask yourself, how will you feel next week if you don't do this now?" (One student wrote himself a reminder of how stressed he felt right after he had to scramble to finish a paper the night before it was due. He gave the coach a copy and asked to be reminded to read this periodically.)

Issue:	**Planning and prioritizing**

Understanding the Issue

The need for planning and prioritizing one's actions arises dozens of times a day. Most of us take these necessary skills so much for granted that we have no idea when or how we developed them. Webster's College Dictionary defines these important skills as follows:

> **{ Planning:** Developing a scheme or method of acting in advance or having in mind an intention **}**

> **{ Prioritizing:** Arranging or doing something in order of priority (having the right to precede others) **}**

For individuals without disabilities, using one's thoughts to plan and prioritize tasks seems to happen almost magically and effortlessly. While we may have attended some workshops or courses that touched on these skills, most people have probably just figured them out or learned from watching others. We simply expect ourselves and others to deliberately determine what we intend to do with our time and, on the whole, to carry out our intentions successfully.

Before attending college, most young adults have had to develop their planning and prioritizing skills and strategies to some extent. Increased academic expectations, social life, extracurricular activities, family chores, and part-time jobs have probably forced most teens to develop some system of managing time to make sure they get things done. However, for most entering freshmen, college is the first time their success really depends on total mastery of their ability to plan and prioritize. College will force students to stretch these abilities in ways they never imagined. There are so many possible experiences vying for a college student's time. They quickly learn that "going with the flow" and just letting life happen is a nonproductive strategy, given the many deadlines and activities they must learn to juggle. Students must learn to keep track of the various experiences of their college life, like going to class, studying, attending interesting social and group activities, social time with friends, and doing chores like laundry, paying bills, etc. "Burning the candle at both ends" is one way many college students choose initially to handle this new, stimulating life. But sooner of later, every college student needs to find a healthier, more effective system of scheduling their time and deciding which activities are most important to do on any given day. Knowing that developing these skills and strategies is a challenge for many students, campus counseling offices, learning skills centers, and student health programs frequently offer a host of workshops and one-to-one services to aid students with time management and the challenge of adjusting to college life.

Why do college students with AD/HD have difficulty with planning and prioritizing?

The answer to this question may be rather obvious by now. People with AD/HD often find thinking before acting and thinking long enough to critically evaluate their priorities an extremely difficult and sometimes impossible task. In fact, many students with this disability report that they tend to get into action without much deliberation about what is the most important thing to do and how best to do it. Some students with AD/HD report that they prefer to live life in a much more spontaneous manner, without a plan. Other students who want to use their time efficiently and make a schedule for themselves repeatedly fail when they try to follow their schedule. Constant failure is discouraging and many conclude that it is not worth the bother to plan or prioritize at all. As one college student with AD/HD lamented, "I use to say I hated planning and prioritizing and anyone who did these things couldn't be my friend. But the truth was that I was afraid to do either of these things. I couldn't trust my own ability to recall or figure out what my priorities were and I just couldn't keep my mind in planning mode long enough to create a workable plan. I'd get distracted, bored, or just need to do something active. Planning is passive and I hate passive!" So various elements of AD/HD conspire to produce what appears to be the free-will choice to chronically procrastinate, followed by last-minute panic and desperate attempts to catch up.

Many college students with AD/HD have lived their entire lives just "letting life happen," a skill that many workaholics and more scheduled people wish they could develop. While living in the moment can be viewed as a strength, if this is one's exclusive mode of functioning it can also cause problems.College students with AD/HD are not consistently able to plan effectively because they cannot engage in the cognitive processes of planning and prioritizing tasks. Some complain of being stuck in the nonproductive cycle of periods of being on top of things; planning, prioritizing, using a calendar and keeping to a schedule, followed by times when their lives reel out of control. Many students indicate that they have never been able to establish the habit of deliberately thinking about how to manage their daily lives. Consequently, some college students with AD/HD have lost hope of life ever being significantly different than it is; and worse yet, their ability to make progress is hampered by emotional scars and wounds from past failures in this area. Most discover the hard way in college that they *must* modify their go-with-the-flow or last minute approach to life, but have no faith in their own ability to make this happen.

Coaching can be a lifesaver in helping college students with AD/HD deal with their weaknesses in planning and prioritizing. In fact, helping the college student overcome these weaknesses is what coaching is essentially all about. Unlike traditional, canned approaches to time and task management, coaching enables the college student with AD/HD to develop ways to plan and prioritize that are uniquely matched to his or her own needs, talents, and shortcomings. Since the coach's primary mode of communication is to ask questions, the student is given ample opportunity to explore different systems and strategies, and to experiment to determine which might be helpful. Coaching provides a nonjudgmental relationship where the student is allowed to try out and develop these thinking skills, secure in the knowledge that the coach will be there to catch anything that is missed. Sometimes, that security is all the student needs in order to take the risk of focusing on one thing at a time. In fact, many times the coach simply serves as a "witness" who just sits next to the student while he or she engages in the process of planning.

Students with AD/HD also report that they typically don't look at a calendar and actually "see" where they are in time, even though they know this is important to do. Without the coaching relationship to encourage regular, brief periods of sitting still and thinking about their lives, many students report that they would never actually think much about the passage of time, never mind the layout of a plan for a long-term project, assignment, or exam. Through the use of questioning, the coach tries to increase the likelihood that the college student with AD/HD will analyze tasks, determine workable time schedules for task completion, and get better at sticking to those schedules.

Ultimately, the power of coaching lies in the fact that it allows students with AD/HD to develop the planning strategies that meet their own unique needs and are more likely to be used regularly. Published calendars and day-planning systems may never meet the needs of some students with AD/HD. Such students can become creative in the coaching relationship and discover that they can generate new systems and techniques of recording plans and schedules that really work for them. Similarly, the coaching relationship can help students form the habit of *using* the planning tool of their choice, whether it is a day-planner they made or purchased or an electronic organizer that has been sitting in a box unopened. Living through the difficult process of deliberate habit formation is something many college students with AD/HD say they could never achieve on their own.

Addressing the Issue

The coach can help the student:

1 **Determine his preferences for planning.**

Examples:

- Determine how often the student wants to meet and the period for which the student wants to plan. For most students, planning for a whole week is overwhelming and while they may like making a weekly priority list, they frequently want to break this up into daily plans. Initially, some students only want to think about blocks of time as small as one hour, a half-day, or a day. Others want to plan for a portion of a week, perhaps two days at a time.

- Discuss how the student prefers to plan during coaching sessions. For example, some students want the coach to simply be a "witness" present in the room while they silently plan; others prefer to talk aloud and have the coach listen while they write up their plans and think out priorities. Others want to talk while the coach writes up the plan.

2 **Develop external structures to encourage planning and prioritizing by creating and selecting planning tools that are personalized to the student's needs.**

Example:

- Many AD/HD students can be creative with Post-it notes, their own hands, small sheets of paper, pieces of note book paper, small spiral notebooks, white boards, voice mail, email etc. Let the student experiment with different ways of recording plans and appointments and discover what really helps, and thus are more likely to use.

3 **Engineer the environment to encourage effective planning and prioritizing.**

Examples:

- Ask the student if he or she would like to be accountable to the coach for daily planning. This may take the form of calling the coach or emailing daily plans or actually scheduling frequent coaching contacts at a consistent time. The aim is to promote the habit of thinking out the day.

- Build in a few minutes at the start of each coaching contact to read the student's course syllabi and map out the assignments for the upcoming week. Look ahead for long-term assignments and encourage the student to analyze the small steps toward completing these.

- Put all big assignments and tests on a monthly calendar and display this prominently in the student's apartment or room. Some students prefer that the coach keep these calendars and want to refer to them only during coaching meetings.

- Encourage the student to ask a friend to be a planning coach who listens to daily plans.

4 **Develop internal structures that promote planning and prioritizing. The coach can model this by asking questions.**

Planning:

- What absolutely has to get done today?

- What small steps can you take to help you get that task done? Which small step will you take first?

- Does it matter when you do each task?

- What might interfere with you following your plan? (Encourage the student to acknowledge the enormous variety of distractions and obstacles, both positive and negative that can throw one off course.) How can you deal with these distractions and/or overcome these barriers?

- What might help you follow your plan?

Prioritizing:

- What are all the things you need to get done during a given time period (like a half day, one day, two days, and a week)?

- Which of these tasks absolutely has to get done today because of an imminent deadline?

- Which of these have to get done because not doing them will make it much harder to meet a deadline later on?

- Which are things you feel like doing but can really wait?

5 **Encourage the internalization of the questions that promote planning and prioritizing by eventually agreeing to have the student be more active during the session.**

Examples:

- The student can generate his or her own list of questions to promote planning. Make these visible during sessions to help the student be more independent during planning activities

- Have the student design a worksheet that can be used during planning and prioritizing.

- Record questions on posters, bookmarks, or other signs that can be prominently displayed to remind about the cognitive process used for planning and prioritizing.

6 Use rewards/consequences to help develop the habit of daily planning and prioritizing.

Examples:
- Have the student agree to pay the coach a fine for not doing a daily plan. The student agrees to send accumulated money to his or her least favorite charity.

- Make an appointment to do planning at a coffee shop or during a lunch meeting with a friend.

- Follow planning with a favorite activity like surfing the Internet, working out at the gym, or walking the dog.

7 Make planning a habit by grouping it with an already existing habit.

Examples:
- Plan immediately after a particular meal each day.

- Plan before bedtime.

- Use time between classes for planning.

8 Increase awareness of the value of planning and prioritizing.

Examples:
- Have the student reflect on the differences he or she experiences on days when planning has occurred and days when it has not.

- Make a list of all the real life consequences of planning vs. not planning

9 To become increasingly independent at planning and prioritizing.

Examples:

- Have the student agree to slowly fade the coach's involvement during planning time in meetings.

- Once appropriate strategies have been developed, start having the student plan in a different room, away from the coach. Then have the student and coach debrief how the planning process went.

- Have the student attend the coaching session, but sit alone to plan and then leave a copy of the plan for the coach to review.

Making decisions and solving problems

Understanding the Issue

Freshmen must be able to make good decisions and solve problems effectively if they are going to transition successfully to college and continue to have a positive undergraduate experience. Most parents experience some anxiety about how their young person will cope with the freedom and temptations that college life offers. All parents hope that their sons or daughters will succeed in college without enduring any major life crises. The moment that parents say "good-byes," leaving the student alone in the dorm, the need to become an independent decision-maker and problem-solver surfaces. There are academic issues like what classes to take and when to take them, when to study, whether to drop a class, how to talk to a professor, what major to select, what topic to choose for a paper, how to study for a test, where to study and with whom, whether to attend class or not?

At times, students may encounter more serious decisions or problems related to their academic life, such as: should they ask another student to help them write a paper even when this violates the honor code, is it OK to consult the fraternity and sorority files for papers and tests; or should they join others in cheating during an exam? Life outside of the classroom presents a host of new and equally problematic situations, some that are minor and others that could have a major impact on the young person's life. Issues like: when to wake up and when to go to bed, how to decorate the dorm room, what style of fashion to wear, what to eat, whether to go to church, how to handle a roommate problem, how to manage money, pay bills, be responsible with a credit card, whether to pledge a sorority or fraternity or join a particular club, whether to get a tattoo, pierce a body part or color one's hair, whether to be sexually active, use drugs, or indulge in alcohol. The potential list of decisions and problematic situations a student could face at college is endless and could frighten even the most trusting parents about sending their young adults to college.

Becoming an independent decision-maker and problem-solver is one of the most important tasks that all human beings must face. This learning process is difficult for all individuals as they move toward adulthood. Probably anyone who has attended college has stories about the mistakes and crazy things that they did because they lacked a well-developed decision-making or problem-solving process. Even if college wasn't part of an individual's life experience, few people get to adulthood without having an embarrassing moment, having made some mistakes, or without having several skeletons hidden in their closets—all of which may be related to faulty decision making and/or problem-solving skills.

Consider for a moment what it takes to engage in these important thinking processes. First, we must suspend action and engage in reflection and notice the warning signs that a problem is evolving or an important decision has presented itself. It is important that we identify the presence of a problem or an important decision before time runs out and the situation is at a crisis level. Surely, we may have strong emotions that must be managed so we can be objective and think clearly rather than react. This is no easy task and we may stay stuck in nonproductive emotions for a while before we can move on. Once we become unstuck, we can generate our options. Sometimes, we need help expanding our vision to see that there are more than the limited options we have generated. Either/or thinking can limit us, and friends or other support people play an important role in helping us, consider other options. It may be too hard on our own to brainstorm freely without immediately criticizing the options we generate or are given. Then the decision-making process must begin and we have to evaluate the options based on a variety of factors: past experience, our values, preferences, and our educated guesses about what might happen if we implement each option. The selection process is difficult, to say the least. Our heart may be cueing us to one path and our head to another. We all must develop some method of weighing pros and cons of the alternatives. Eventually, we must make a choice about what path to pursue and develop a plan to implement it that is workable. Like so many other higher level thinking skills, most of us take our decision-making and problem-solving abilities for granted. Typically, we have not had formal instruction in these skills; instead, instruction is sort of a "learn as you go" endeavor. We improve in these important thinking skills throughout our lives from observing others, getting their advice at key moments, and productively extracting the lessons from our past decisions that went awry. Luckily, with maturity and experience, most people develop a productive method for inhibiting impulsive actions and selecting the best option to handle the endless decisions and problems that are a constant part of daily life.

In most cases, freshmen come to college with ample practice using these cognitive abilities and already have strategies to stop and think carefully, to analyze a problem, and to consider the alternatives *before* deciding upon a plan of action. Most will have little difficulty recognizing when an important decision needs to be made or when a potentially significant problem is developing, and will openly seek the advice of trusted support people, including their parents, and carefully scrutinize the situation. Without any major impairment to hamper their thinking, most freshmen are likely to learn from their past and alter their decision-making and problem-solving skills to adjust to the expectations of college life.

It is widely accepted that individuals with AD/HD can experience the most disabling effects of their disability when they attempt to engage in decision-making and problem-solving. Like other cognitive skills (planning, prioritizing) quality problem-solving and decision-making are dependent on the individual's ability to engage in reflection for a period of time and to delay action. Using these higher-level thinking skills may be very difficult and nearly impossible for some college students with AD/HD. Since these important skills typically are not taught directly and must be acquired through observation of self and others, it is likely that some college students with AD/HD may not have developed these abilities to a level that is matched to their intellectual potential. Others, however, may have strengths in these areas and have excelled in life because of these abilities.

Once focused on a problem, individuals with AD/HD may be able to generate a host of novel options for its resolution. However, many report not being able to stop moving, talking, or thinking long enough to fully evaluate a decision, analyze and think through how to solve a particular problem, and/or how to follow through on what they think is the best plan of action. Staying focused on an idea without being sidetracked by other thoughts or stimuli in the environment may be a struggle. Similarly, inhibiting action to allow for introspection may be equally challenging. As one young man indicated, "Before I know it, I have made a decision, even when I have a gut feeling that what I am doing is wrong. It's almost like I can't stop myself from reacting in the moment and I agree to something that I later regret. It never fails, and usually I am upset with myself for buying something I didn't need or doing something I am sorry for. The weird thing is I can go out and do the same thing again the next day." As this young man's comments reveal, the pattern of faulty decision-making and problem-solving can become chronic because the student may have difficulty productively analyzing past mistakes, so that he or she can learn from them.

Impulsivity can also prevent an individual from gathering all the important facts during the problem definition stage, resulting in faulty perceptions about the situation. An example involves a young man who started his coaching session very distraught. "I am failing my Biology class," he said, "and the deadline to drop the class has passed. Can you get me out of the class?" Rather than determining how to help him drop the class, the coach knew, from past experience, to spend more time defining the problem. He asked, "What facts do you have that make you feel certain you are failing?" This question led to the realization that the student didn't know for sure if he was failing. He had received several grades that appeared to be low, but he was unsure how to interpret the professor's grading scale. After talking with the coach, the student "saw" that he needed more information before jumping to the conclusion that the class needed to be dropped. He called the professor and discovered that he had a C- in the class. The professor offered to meet with him to go over any concepts that were confusing and causing him to feel like a failure.

Some college students with AD/HD report being immobilized when faced with an important decision or a significant problem. Some share that they get overwhelmed because although they see all the options available, they can't seem to prioritize among them. Others report seeing the possible negative ramifications of various options all too clearly, so they get "stuck" thinking about all the things that could go wrong. Sometimes, a student's past history of poor problem-solving or making "bad" decisions causes an emotional block, and students describe the fact that their thoughts are spinning with feelings, judgements and worries that make objective problem-solving difficult, if not impossible. "I just don't think of the questions to ask to stop myself from reacting emotionally and to start thinking about what my options are," one student with AD/HD stated in a frustrated tone.

Other students indicate that even when they try to think through a decision or engage in problem-solving, they may have trouble freely generating options and further difficulty evaluating their options objectively. One young woman said, "Not being realistic about how a decision will really affect me is the main problem I have in making decisions. So, if I try to decide if I should take five or six classes, I tend to gloss over the facts about how much time I will really need to spend studying and preparing for six classes versus five. Before actually being in the situation, I have this pattern of minimizing how hard things will be. I seem to totally forget how stressed I felt in the past. I tell myself, glibly, I can handle it! I am also very stubborn and I don't take advice well. So, if other people try to get me to see the truth about the choice I am making, I tend to resist what they are saying. When reality hits, I am freaked out because it seems too late to change the situation and I remember at the wrong time that I really can't handle it." This young woman's story also highlights an additional issue that can hamper some students with AD/HD from capitalizing on the good advice of advisors, friends, and family members. Some students honestly indicate that they are independent learners who prefer to learn from their own experience rather than from the advice of other people. As this young woman points out, for some individuals with AD/HD, the more someone suggests avoiding an option, the more appealing the option becomes.

Finally, the deficits college students with AD/HD demonstrate in independent decision-making and problem-solving may also be related to their lack of practice. Some students report that teachers and parents were intimately involved in helping them in the past. Consequently, they may have had limited opportunities to develop their own problem-solving abilities because others told them what to do and what not to do. Others report that many problems were avoided by well-meaning parents or teachers who provided so much structure and support that the need to make a decision never arose and problems were eliminated or "nipped in the bud."

One of the most valuable contributions the coaching relationship can provide to college students with AD/HD is the awareness that there are options to their current habits and behaviors. Coaching can help the student become more deliberate about how they deal with the problems and decisions they encounter on a daily basis. Although some students may seek coaching because they know they have limitations in the higher-level thinking skills, others may lack this level of self-understanding. Some may not realize that the behaviors they are describing that cause stress result from their disability and, even more importantly, are the result of choices they have made. Students may view their chronic patterns of procrastination or frequent episodes of being sidetracked when trying to complete a task, getting stuck in hyperfocus, as well as their tendency to respond impulsively to decisions and problems, as, "this is what I do and have always done." Many students judge themselves harshly for engaging in these behaviors, seeing how they clearly cause havoc, at times, in their lives. Because AD/HD is a neurologically based condition, it truly is very difficult, and for some individuals with AD/HD, nearly impossible for them to stop and observe themselves in the moment, to evaluate the decision and to later engage in productive retrospection. Consequently, they may never have seen that there is another way. Even when they have seen their options, some may have a long history of failed attempts at improving their decision-making or refining their problem-solving ability. This trail of failure can result in a belief system that change isn't possible and a sense of hopelessness about changing one's fate may prevail. Coaching can raise awareness about habitual patterns of making decisions or dealing with problems and provide hope that things can be different.

By forming a partnership with a coach, progress can be made in the development of the student's decision-making and problem-solving skills. The coaching relationship can offer a comfortable setting for the student to explore how AD/HD gets in the way of decision-making and problem-solving without the fear of being judged or criticized. All too frequently, students report having heard negative remarks from parents, teachers, and other adults commenting on how poorly a decision was made or the ineffective methods used to solve a problem. "My entire life, people have said things like, 'What were you thinking when you made this decision or were you even thinking at all,'" one young woman confided with tears in her eyes. "It feels so good to talk to someone about my difficulties making decisions and not feel totally ashamed."

The coach can be invaluable in helping students by providing the self-talk necessary to promote quality problem-solving and decision-making. The coach models the questions that stimulate this type of thinking and can actually compensate for the student's deficiencies with these cognitive skills. Hopefully, college students with AD/HD will begin to use these skills independently as a result of the repeated modeling and practice that occurs during coaching sessions. The coaching relationship can allow the student to observe him or herself and uncover the need to address a potential problem before it is too late. The coach's questions can allow students the opportunity to use their creativity to see options and take the time to evaluate each alternative more critically. One young man told his coach, "When I'm talking with you about a decision or problem, I know I will stay focused on one idea and take the time to think more clearly about everything. If I am by myself, I just don't seem able to do this. Before I know it, I am getting up doing something else or my mind switches to some other issue."

The student can also guide the coach on how to handle times when emotions are blocking clear thinking about a decision or problem. With the student's permission, the coach can give feedback like "This seems like a time when emotions are in the way." The coaching relationship can increase the likelihood that the student deals productively with these emotions. When appropriate, the coach can help the student discern that emotions are a significant barrier to productive thinking and that the student needs to "take this situation to your therapist," or be referred to a therapist to deal with these emotional issues.

Addressing the Issue

The coach can help the student:

1 **Promote awareness of the events that led to the problem being discussed.**

Example:

- When the student is describing a situation that had caused problems, the coach can ask if the student thinks it might be helpful to take a moment to analyze what events led to this situation. If the student's emotions are running high, he or she may not want to or be able to engage in objective analysis of the past. The coach can pose questions like: "What are the events that led to this situation?" "What did you do that helped?" "What decisions did you make that may have contributed to the problem?" "What kind of thinking did you engage in when you were dealing with this problem or decision?" "If you could replay this situation, what other choices might you make?" "What type of thinking might be helpful?" "How can your knowledge about this situation be useful in the future?"

2 **Promote awareness that options exist.**

Examples:

- In response to the student's comments that reveal that he or she feels like there is no other option ("I just can't stop myself from procrastinating," or "being side-tracked," or "acting impulsively"), the coach can ask questions that promote seeing options like: "If a friend came to you and said what you are saying now, how would you respond?" "Let's pretend for a moment that you could stop yourself, what would that look like?"

- Ask the student to think of a time when he or she did not engage in the behavior being discussed (e.g. procrastination, getting sidetracked, reacting impulsively, etc.). Ask questions like: "What was different about that time?" "What choices led to a different outcome?"

- When a student is stuck seeing no or limited options ask: "What other options are there?" "Would you like me to share some other options I've seen other students use?"

3 Establish the relationship.

Example:

- The student can design the coaching relationship to focus on monitoring issues related to problem-solving and decision-making. One student asked that her coach take a few minutes at the start of each meeting to reflect upon whether any problems or important decisions that need attention might be surfacing in her life. This would then allow the coaching session to focus on these issues. Whenever a student discusses a problem or a decision during a session, the coach should explicitly ask the student what role he or she should play during the discussion of the problem. Students may indicate that they just want the coach to listen and allow them the opportunity to think aloud. Others may want the coach to pose questions to make sure that the issue is being critically evaluated. Some may prefer the coach to be more directive in guiding their thinking.

4 Use questions to promote reflection.

Example:

- The coach can ask the student questions to promote more careful thought—Asking broad questions can help students draw on past experiences or simply use their creativity to focus on the issue at hand. Questions similiar to the ones listed here can encourage students to stop and think: "What have you done in the past to help you make decisions?" "What will help you make this decision?" "What facts do you need to gather to help you make your decision?" "What options do you have?" "How can you choose among them?" These questions can help ensure that the student will be more thoughtful.

5 Develop external structures to promote thinking objectively about problems and decisions.

Example:

- Each student can identify tools that might prevent impulsive responding and increase the likelihood of careful thought. Some students prefer to make personalized signs to post at key places in their environment. Others may choose to create "rules" for problem-solving and decision-making that can be both prompts to slow down and guides for thinking. Trusted friends can also be called upon to prompt thinking through decisions carefully and to ensure that quality problem-solving occurs. Students can prevent unwanted nagging and help by telling friends what to say that would be helpful.

6 Develop internal structures to promote thinking objectively about problems and decisions.

Example:

- Many times problem-solving is blocked by thoughts that prompt action or emotional thoughts versus logical thinking. Thoughts like, "There's no way this will work out," or "I have to know right now" will inhibit careful thinking. Students can work with their coaches to identify productive self-talk that might alter their thinking in a positive direction. Mantras like "OK, now slow down and think this through," or "What are all my options for dealing with this?" can serve to move a person into the realm of critical thinking.

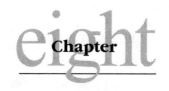

Chapter eight

PERSONAL SKILLS— ISSUES FOR COLLEGE STUDENTS WITH AD/HD

What is it all about?

AD/HD coaching is wholistic and helps students to examine all aspects of their lives, how they live it, the choices they make, and the effects these choices have on the quality of their life. Some students with AD/HD may not see the importance of exploring these more personal issues and might only want to focus on improving their grades. However, coaching is much more than simply helping students obtain goals and improve academic performance. By working with a coach, students have an opportunity to explore and understand how and why they behave the way they do through the lens of their AD/IID. Coaching is about more than helping students with AD/HD get things done. Coaching helps to develop self-understanding and self-acceptance, through promoting self-observation. Not all students are ready or able to partake in this process of self-discovery. In some cases, the student might be better off working with another type of professional—who use more traditional approaches to learning strategy instruction. Additionally, other issues might crop up in the student's personal life that might require the help of a psychiatrist or another mental health professional. A coach is not equipped or qualified to handle all life issues that arise during coaching, but rather is trained to make referrals to appropriate professionals to handle issues out of their area of expertise.

Because of the frequent contact a coach has with a client, coaches are in the unique position to make observations about how students live on a daily basis and to raise their awareness about areas of concern or the introspection they need for improvement. By helping the student engage in self-observation, coaches can help generate ways to better manage stress, identify internal tapes that block progress, and establish obtainable goals, and identify nonproductive patterns.

College is about becoming independent, exploring one's own identity, and growing and learning from one's experiences. However, what happens when a student's ability to learn from his/her own mistakes is compromised or delayed? This is one of the major issues for students with AD/HD—many times they keep repeating the same mistakes not knowing how to implement strategies or to self-correct. Learning to be a good self-observer is a skill that needs time and practice to develop. With this skill in place, a student with AD/HD can be in a better position to identify and manage stress, set obtainable goals, and learn ways to replace self-defeating patterns with healthier ones.

How does coaching help?

Being aware of what personal issue gets in the way of progress is very important. Coaching helps to students with AD/HD slow down so they can think before they act. The relationship with a coach is also a safe place to receive feedback about one's behavior and about one's choices. Often, consequences of actions or decisions are not well thought out or even considered by students with AD/HD. By working with a coach, students with AD/HD are able to verbalize thoughts and ideas and walk through actions in advance. Ultimately, by practicing the skill of self-observation, a student with AD/HD can develop better judgment and, most of all, start to develop more confidence to become a more reliable and responsible adult.

It would be a mistake to measure students—AD/HD or not—solely on the basis of their academic performance. However, this is the gauge by which most students are measured or measure themselves in academic arenas. Coaching aims to help students with AD/HD look beyond these measures to develop life skills as well as improve their academic performance.

For students with AD/HD, success in college and life beyond academia lies in their ability to understand and accept themselves and their disability, and to learn to live a more balanced and organized life. By focusing on personal issues, coaching can facilitate growth in these critical areas.

Issue:

Negative self-talk

Understanding the Issue

In his book, "Taming Your Gremlin," Richard D. Carson talks about the power that negative tapes play in our lives and how they work to sabotage our happiness. Often by the time young adults with AD/HD reach college, they have already developed an extensive repertoire of negative self-talk full of "I can'ts" and "If onlys." These negative tapes reflect feelings about how their disability has been seen by others as either willful or a character flaw. Unfortunately, these tapes can be deeply rooted and significantly influence the student's belief about what he or she can and cannot do. Even worse, the negative thoughts chip away at the ability to develop self-worth, distorting self-image and damaging self-esteem. It is no wonder that adults with AD/HD are at greater risk for developing coexisting psychological and emotional disorders such as: depression, anxiety, obsessive compulsive disorders, drug and alcohol dependence, and eating disorders.

Addressing the Issue

The coach can help the student:

Label it. Help students identify their negative tapes, by becoming aware of what they say to themselves, and when the tapes start to play. Some coaches call these tapes "Gremlins" (as described in Richard Carson's book). Carson suggests that each person make the "Gremlin" concrete by giving them a name, a shape, a form, and/or a color. Coaches can quickly point out these sabotaging tapes to students and help shut them off. For example, a coach can say, "There goes Fred again! He's convincing you that you are going to fail your test!" Using this technique, a coach will be better able to help students identify these defeating thoughts and "reprogram" them to more positive messages.

Plan for the attack. Once a coach knows when and what makes these negative tapes play, he can help the student actually plan for them. The student can be encouraged to program the coach to remind him or her of these situations, and thus encourage techniques that counteract the "Gremlin" ahead of time.

Notice his language. Part of learning positive self-talk is to take notice of the language an individual uses to talk about himself. Coaches can encourage students to look out for when they use negative terms and descriptions about themselves. Students may find it helpful to write these messages down, and then make a list of new phrases—positive ones—to replace them. Students can set a goal of using at least one positive phrase a day so that these new positive thoughts can become part of their daily language.

Externalize to internalize. Encourage students to practice thinking, saying, and writing positive things about themselves. Have them use their environment to reinforce these affirmations by posting written reminders or symbols. For example, they could hang a big plus sign or a smiley face on their bathroom mirror so they will be reminded to practice positive self-talk.

Use a tracking system. Students can be accountable to their coach for a specified amount of time (two or more days) to keep track of their negative thoughts. Suggest they put a hash mark on a piece of paper (or their hand) each time they have one of these thoughts. Once they have tracked the number of negative thoughts per day (i.e., 57), coaches might encourage them try to create the same number (57) of positive thoughts. This not only makes it fun, but will give them a more tangible, conscious way to "see" how they think and help them alter defeating patterns.

Seek help from other medical or mental health professionals. At times, negative self-talk can be symptomatic of more serious psychological illness. Students need to be referred to a psychiatrist, therapist, or counselor when their negative self-talk doesn't change after focusing on this during coaching or if they have a co-existing emotional disorder that is impacting on their functioning.

Issue:	
	Managing stress

Understanding the Issue

A key to managing stress is recognizing it, knowing its effects, and identifying the causes. So often we hear students with AD/HD say, "I did not realize I was getting sick" or "I totally forgot I had a test in the morning when I decided to stay up all night." Overcommitting, not getting enough sleep, and not evaluating consequences all take part in creating stressful situations. The hidden challenge of the college experience for ALL students is that of learning one's limits without parental guidance and being able to set appropriate boundaries. Students with AD/HD often don't learn from their mistakes and have trouble setting boundaries. To make matters worse, stress in and of itself, oftentimes, is used as a tool to propel students with AD/HD into action. For example, waiting until the last minute to complete a paper or study for an exam can give the student with AD/HD the conditions needed to take action. AD/HD and stress, at some level may need to coexist, but if not managed correctly, can quickly become overwhelming and lead to a host of serious problems.

Many college students don't know what it takes to be healthy and even if they do, they forget to engage in good health practices as a means of stress prevention. Most new freshmen have taken the healthy home cooked meals and their parents reminders "to get some sleep" for granted. It is only after the fact, when they become sick that they take notice and begin to make changes in how they manage stress and care for themselves. However, students with AD/HD are less likely to learn from the past.

A less obvious cause of stress for students with AD/HD is the fact that they are operating out of areas of weakness. College demands that they constantly do what is difficult for them to do: sit still, listen, and engage in passive activities. Students with AD/HD can become worn down by overcompensating and not understand how to correct the situation. A coach can help identify a student's preferred mode of learning and help develop strategies to avoid drawing on his or her weaknesses and to promote practices that are better matched to his or her strengths.

Clearly coaching is not a cure-all for helping students deal with their stress. If a student's stress becomes unmanageable or if he or she is experiencing depression, changes in eating habits, panic attacks, or insomnia, he or she should be referred to a physician or other medical or mental health professionals.

Addressing the Issue

The coach can help the student:

Practice extreme self-care. This means developing a routine for adequate sleep, healthy eating, drinking lots of water, exercising regularly and having periods of rest and relaxation. Coaches can encourage the creation of a check-in system so that students can follow through on these things. Creating healthy habits can help students keep up their energy reserves and thus be less likely to be affected by stress.

Exercise. Encourage students to enlist a "no excuses" attitude with themselves when it comes to exercise. There is ample evidence about the positive effects of exercise on reducing stress, anxiety, and depression. Even short bouts of exercise (like jumping rope or a brisk 10 minute walk) have been shown to reduce stress levels. Coaches can help students learn not to let anything stop them by encouraging them to get up and move when they are feeling anxious, as well as sticking to their exercise goals.

Plan ahead. If students know that certain situations are stressful —for example, writing papers—have them program the coach, to remind them of this fact well in advance of the due dates. Typical strategies might be exercising more and getting more sleep, or canceling any extracurricular obligations around those dates. This helps students to protect themselves against the up-coming stress. The fact that the stress does not catch them off guard is powerful in and of itself.

Listen to his or her body. Coaches can help students try to identify what happens to their body when they get stressed. Do they clench their jaw? Bite their nails? Tighten their back? Get an upset stomach? If students become aware of the "early warning signs" of stress, they can avoid their old patterns. Students can program the coach to help them observe themselves by asking questions like, "How much are you biting your nails lately?" "Has your stomach been upset this week?" This will help students to pay more attention to what their body is telling them so they can take measures to reduce stress before it becomes toxic.

Use strengths. To further lower stress, coaches can work with students to identify their preferred learning style and where their strengths lie. Coaches can "free" students to be creative and use strength-based strategies, even if they are seen as unconventional (like dictating a paper, or listening to books on tape).

Use powerful images. Coaches can encourage students to use an image to express how they feel. One student said that when he was stressed, he felt like a wild octopus frantically trying to do everything at the same time, tentacles flying in every direction, out of control. To help him get more grounded in these situations, the coach then came up with the image of an elephant, slowing walking with its huge, heavy feet, taking very purposeful steps. When he felt stressed and out-of-control, he could quickly and easily grab onto the image of the elephant. The coach would ask him questions like, "How can you be more elephant-like this week?" The use of images is a powerful tool in helping to change behavior and "re-set" mental states.

Encourage periods of relaxation. Many students with AD/HD are always "on the go," rushing and doing. Coaches can encourage students to explore how doing nothing and being still at various points throughout the day can reduce their stress level.

Seek out campus resources for various stress management and centering activities. While aerobic exercise can help the body deal with stress, these activities may not center the body, the mind, and the spirit. Activities like karate, yoga, tai-chi, meditation and prayer can be beneficial at promoting calmness and centering. Many religious organizations on campus have groups to promote daily prayer and meditation. In addition, most student health centers and recreation centers sponsor programs on developing these healthy habits. Coaches can encourage students to become aware of these resources and use them.

> **Issue:**
>
> ### Establishing realistic goals

Understanding the Issue

Oftentimes, students with AD/HD set themselves up for failure by thinking they can accomplish more than is possible in a given amount of time. This can happen for a variety of reasons. AD/HD distorts an individual's ability to measure time. If one's sense of time is off, planning anything realistically can be next to impossible. Also, many students with AD/HD are able to "see" the project in its entirety and "see" what the end product looks like. Unfortunately, with this ability comes a drawback; an inability to break the big goal into its component parts and a sequential set of steps. Many consequences ensue from this, for example, leaving things to the last minute because there is a false sense of what actually needed to be done. The student with AD/HD can get completely overwhelmed when trying to break down the big picture. The end result is usually the same—not getting work done and/or undergoing a lot of stress and panic. Part of the charm of students with AD/HD is that they live in the moment—they don't necessarily get lost living in the future. They act impulsively, bite off more than they can chew, overcommit, and end up with a classic case of indigestion!

A coaching partnership can help students engage in frequent reality checks. By talking things through with a coach, notions or ideas can be more grounded. A coach also can help students learn to create time lines and break large or long-range projects into smaller chunks.

Addressing the Issue

A coach can help the student:

Be realistic. Take what a student thinks he or she wants to accomplish and either divide it or multiply it by two. For example, if he or she thinks it will take four hours to complete a paper, plan for eight hours. If he or she wants to exercise one hour each day, plan for a half hour. Encourage the student to plan out all goals and tasks with estimated times using the above method. He or she can learn to block out these hours on the weekly schedule. Keeping track of the actual amount of time the tasks take to do. This will help students become more realistic about their goals.

Create awareness of "self-sleezing." This means to be aware of when one lies to oneself. Encourage students to be honest about these patterns. This concept is more profound than simply fooling oneself. It takes place when an individual is completely convinced he or she WILL do something, and then doesn't. For example, many students wait until evening to study, the time when their roommates are home and starting to party. Or they commit to tasks for a group project when they don't have the time to complete them. Often, they don't even realize they are lying to themselves or to others. But the end result is always the same, the student falls short of the goal and builds a "trail of failure" instead of a "trail of success."

Make it part of a natural routine. Many students think that if they set aside all day Saturday and Sunday to study everything will be okay. Unfortunately, this type of scheduling only leads to getting overwhelmed, feeling defeated, and not studying. Goals need to fit in the rhythm of their lives, otherwise they won't get accomplished. To do this the coach needs to get a clear sense of what the student does on a daily and weekly basis. What recurring weekly commitments does he or she have besides classes? Help students map out what a typical week looks like to see their time, and isolate places where goals could naturally fit into their schedule. For example, going to the library for two hours in between afternoon classes, or exercising on mornings they have a late class. Have them mark these goals on their weekly schedule so that nothing else will take its place. It is important to set the intention and then protect that space. Students can post the weekly template by their computers or other visible places to remind them of their commitments so they will be met.

Introduce the concept of "programming" the coach. It is important for students to know what sidetracks them in their goal attainment. Coaches can work with students to verbalize this and to identify ways to keep them motivated, focused, and true to their goal. Ask students to think about what gets in the way like getting to the library to study is a problem, because they know that going back to their dorm sidetracks them. Get their permission to remind them of this problem by saying. "Remember, if you go back to your dorm, you usually end up hanging out with your friends." By reminding the student of where the potholes in the road are, he or she can better learn to maneuver around them. Because the student gives the coach the right to give the reminder, he or she is more likely to listen.

Create a win-win scenario. Expecting too much too soon is not only unrealistic, but sets people up for failure and leads to abandoning one's goal. Build in flexibility with goals and plan for the unexpected. This way, if students miss one step, they won't feel completely defeated. Help students accommodate for such situations by setting up a minimum and maximum goal for each week. This allows for flexibility, but still holds them to a minimum acceptable standard, for example, exercise a minimum of two times a week and a maximum of four times.

Keep the goal in mind. Perhaps the hardest thing for students with AD/HD is to remember is what their goal is and why it is important. For example, keeping up with weekly assignments is important to doing well in school. Have students write this goal on a card, along with an explanation of why it is important, and post it by their computer or bedside. Create accountability by checking on progress on a regular basis to make sure this goal has not fallen through the cracks.

The eagle vs. the ant view. Establishing realistic goals depends on one's ability to see the big, as well as the small picture. Proper planning requires simultaneously viewing both. Encourage students to post a semester-long calendar by their computer or study station. Have them carry a weekly calendar that also has a daily planner with a to-do list. Have them color code all class due-dates and mark them on the semester-long calendar, as well as the weekly one, so as to see the due-dates at a glance (economics =green; math=red; literature=blue; etc.). This should be done at the beginning of every semester without fail. It is time well spent and prevents getting stuck in either the details or the big picture.

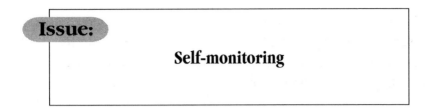

Understanding the Issue

The ability to observe and monitor attention and behavior in the moment is severely challenged for students with AD/HD. Research has indicated that medication can be extremely helpful in mediating impulses so those individuals with AD/HD can slow down long enough to literally "think before they act," and be more conscious of what they are doing. A coach can help students to better understand their AD/HD symptoms and learn and practice ways to self-monitor. Coaches can provide continuous feedback and the structure needed to minimize consequences of this deficit within academic settings.

Coaching is a perfect mechanism for helping students with AD/HD learn how to observe themselves objectively and to consciously redirect themselves to avoid chaos and crisis.

Addressing the Issue

The coach can help the student:

Spy on himself. Encourage students to envision themselves being watched by closed-circuit cameras by "big brother" or a VCR. This metaphor can help give them the distance they need to remove themselves from the moment and to "watch" what they are doing. Encourage students to re-play the film in their head at the end of the day to help them reduce that day's performance. Encourage objective analysis rather than judgement. Questions like, "What did I do that worked?" "What got in my way?" "What will I do differently tomorrow?" can promote objective understanding.

This type of self-monitoring exercise will help them to be more aware of their actions. Students may want to use a calendar or a journal to record these observations or may prefer to email the coach to be accountable for this type of reflection.

Engineer the environment. Encourage students to use timers, pagers, voice-activated reminders, notes posted to themselves, reminders on answering machines, or even messages on a computer screen saver that scrolls, "Are you doing what you planned?" One student learned to stop and evaluate her attention and behavior each time she heard the campus clock chime.

Create structure and accountability. Work with students to identify behaviors and/or actions they want to change. Set up a tangible plan of how they want to go about observing the behavior, what devices and strategies they will use, and when they expect to accomplish their goals. Use check-ins to record observations. This helps to keep the process alive and maintain the goal of reflecting at the forefront of the student's mind.

Encourage asking for feedback. Part of developing the skill of self-monitoring is having an accurate assessment of one's efforts. College courses offer little in terms of feedback. For academic issues, urge students (no matter how painful it is) to meet regularly with professors during office hours to review progress in their course. For other nonacademic issues, such as trying to talk less and listen more in social situations, encourage them to ask for feedback from the coach and/or roommates. Students can compare their own observations to those of others, and alter awareness as needed.

Create "witnesses." Having a "witness" or "monitor" who is present as they work can be an extremely powerful tool in helping students with AD/HD to stay on track. Recent studies have shown that for persons with AD/HD, something as simple as working with a mirror in front of them helped in self-monitoring and improved performance on tasks by 30 percent. Share this information with students and have them use this concept. You might also encourage them to study with a partner or in groups.

> ## Issue:
>
> ## Developing self-awareness

Understanding the Issue

Being self-aware is key to achieving success in one's personal, academic, and professional life. Having an accurate understanding of one's self enables an individual to be proactive in identifying destructive or unwanted behaviors or actions and replacing them with positive ones. The ability to self-correct helps one to grow and change in response to personal and professional environments. Self-awareness allows one to learn from his or her mistakes by developing the necessary skills to avoid past failures and ensure future successes.

In order to change behavior, one must develop a certain level of self-awareness. There are several steps to the process of change. The first step is to recognize that a problem exists. This is also the prerequisite to working with a coach. The second step in both changing behavior and working with a coach is to have a desire and commitment to improving oneself. The third step is to be actively involved in the process by implementing strategies to change unwanted behaviors. The coaching partnership helps to increase self-awareness, and to define and practice strategies that lead to success. Helping students become more aware of their strengths and weaknesses is essential for effective learning. Oftentimes, students with AD/HD, as well as many service providers, approach learning challenges with the mentality of "one strategy fits all." The approach for students with AD/HD has to be an individualized one that plays to the student's strengths. The coaching process helps students with AD/HD explore different learning preferences to discover what works best for them. Operating out of one's strengths, whether one is a visual, auditory, verbal, or kinesthetic learner, is empowering. Identifying and working out of one's strengths increases self-awareness and the chances of academic and personal success.

Perhaps one of the most difficult struggles for persons with AD/HD is that of learning from one's past experiences. The ability to use one's history to identify both positive and negative patterns, and act on that information to promote success or avoid failure, is extremely hard. Some students with AD/HD experience failures and are not even aware of what causes them, while others might know where they got off track, but don't know how to change the circumstances the next time around. Oftentimes, this kind of inability to learn from past mistakes is seen as a character flaw or a lack of desire to change and improve. The symptoms of AD/HD are the culprits of this struggle. Impulsivity, distractibility, and lack of working memory all combine to make it next to impossible for persons with AD/HD to do the necessary reflection that allows them to self-correct. Self-awareness is a key ingredient to combat this issue. By being self-aware, one can identify unwanted behaviors or past patterns and put a plan in place for self-improvement in the future.

Working in partnership with a coach helps students with AD/HD to isolate repeated patterns and replace them with new courses of action. By breaking down the process and identifying where they get stuck, they can better see why they get off track, and determine what they can do about it. Just recognizing that they make the same mistakes over and over again is not enough; taking corrective measures is essential to self-improvement. Coaching provides structure and accountability around the process of change. It helps students to stay involved with the cognitive process long enough to identify and practice strategies and implement a course of action, so that they can independently act before repeating the same mistakes.

Addressing the Issue

The coach can help the student:

"Cement in" the learning process. By working with students, the coach can help them to "cement in" the causes of their mistakes and the solutions needed to remedy them. For this to occur, the coach must be free of judgement and the student must be open to honestly acknowledge his or her role in past mistakes. Assuming both conditions exist, the coach can help the student analyze past situations so he/she can "see" what the mistakes are and how they happened. Recognizing and remembering the mistake is key to stopping the error before it happens and/or implementing a solution. This "cementing in" process is also key to embedding the learning of the solution as well.

Ask for feedback. Many times, students have no awareness of the behaviors they exhibit that are directly related to AD/HD. Self-understanding takes away self-blame and allows students to better understand how their AD/HD impacts them. Suggest a weekly review where you can share your observations. Keeping these discussions at the forefront of the coaching process will help the student to develop more self-awareness.

Stress continued education about AD/HD. Encourage students to learn as much as possible about the causes and effects of AD/HD. Suggest they watch videos, read articles, or surf the web to learn more about AD/HD and how it impacts individuals. Use coaching contacts to discuss what they are learning. Some students find it helpful to keep a log to observe how AD/HD symptoms affect them.

Track progress. Explore with students ways for them to "see" their progress. This will help them to have a sense of accomplishment and keep them motivated. Students can target an unwanted behavior or action and then outline specific measures to combat or change it. For example, getting to bed on time. They can create a chart to track how many nights in a week they make it to bed on time. This will help to remind them of the goal and keep it at the forefront of their mind. It allows them to know how well they are doing and/or what work remains to be done.

Gain knowledge. Work with students to discover what type of learner they are. This can be done by simply helping them reflect on what has worked for them in the past. For example, perhaps making outlines for papers confuses them, but it is obvious that they can see what they want to say in their head, encourage them to "mind-map" or draw out their thoughts before they do an outline? Or perhaps talking out ideas while pacing back and forth in their room helps to clear their head—coaches can give students permission to do what works best for them and stop trying to fit "a square peg into a round hole."

Many times students know certain things work for them, but fight doing them. If the student mentions that quiet study areas are not effective for them, don't encourage them to go to the library. Suggest they go to a coffee shop or a student union where there is a lot of activity, or put on earphones with music. This may seem counterproductive, but if it works for them, don't fight it. If it is clear that they are hyperactive and need to move around, suggest that they not be a passive reader. Trying to sit for hours (something that might work for their peers) will not work for them. A coach can help them acknowledge their need for movement and brainstorm with the student ways to read for short periods of time by taking movement breaks.

Program the coach. The student can program the coach to remind him or her of strengths by asking, "How can you use your strengths to avoid this problem in the future?" This might mean if the student is a visual learner, suggesting that he or she post colorful reminder notes if they tend to forget appointments.

Plan for it. Once students recognize what their mistakes are, coaches can help them plan for them. For example, if they realize that they tend to procrastinate going to the library to study, encourage them to arrange for a friend to call and ask, "Are you headed out the door yet?" Or have them post notes: "Get to the library!" Or have them set an alarm, etc. Continually work with the student to explore ways to catch themselves by anticipating that they WILL procrastinate.

Create rewards. Encourage students to use the information they know about themselves and set up rewards to keep them motivated. For example, if the student knows and admits that she has a hard time completing writing projects, brainstorm ways to set up a reward—for example, after one page is written, have her treat herself to a 15 minute call to a friend. By using information they know about themselves, students can create situations whereby they will feel empowered instead of torn down.

Have periodic checks to compare the past to the present. It can be hard for students to truly see how far they have come. The coach can increase the students' awareness by periodically asking or reminding them to think of how their "old" self would have coped with or handled a situation. This type of discussion can force students to become more aware of what their "new" self is like.

PART
III

CONCLUSION: COACHING— BENEFITS AND LIMITATIONS

nine
Chapter

Coaching—
Benefits and
Limitations

Ask any professional coach, or a college student with AD/HD who has had a coach, and you will hear them extol the many benefits of a coaching relationship. For the college student with AD/HD, coaching can be an important part of a comprehensive treatment program that includes other interventions such as medication, counseling, or therapy. Coaching allows the student to form habits to get things done in a more balanced and organized manner and, in the process, to learn more about what works and doesn't. A coaching relationship can provide students with the tools they need to conquer the symptoms of AD/HD. Above all, coaching can give hope that the future will be different from the past. By helping the student develop a history of success to replace the long history of failure, coaching can improve self-esteem. The following quotes from several students, who have been coached, highlight what students see as the unique contribution coaching has played in their lives.

Benefits for students

Emily, a 23-year-old graduate student with dyslexia and many symptoms of AD/HD:

"Having a coach has made it possible for me to succeed in graduate school. Before I had coaching, my schoolwork and personal life were hopelessly intertwined. I could not see how to plan and prioritize my time between the two. I have learned to prioritize by articulating everything in my life that has to be done without feeling overwhelmed, and then coming up with realistic ways to do it all. Coaching has allowed me to understand the reality of time. Coaching is very different from the counseling/therapy I have had. Both are important for my growth. Instead of dealing with thoughts, feelings and life in the abstract, coaching is about the day-to-day crises I have and how to put the pencil to the calendar to figure out what I am going to do."

Maria, a 19-year-old, second semester sophomore:

"Coaching has been the best thing that ever happened to my study life. I am learning that it isn't impossible to get things done if you know how to break down your time. Even with a crazy college schedule, I can keep things in order. The best part is that I've been able to stop that incessant 'You should be studying' voice— my free time is really free! Knowing that someone else knows what is going on in my life has relieved me of a lot of stress, and I know my schedule better too. My coach helps me maintain a better balance in my life."

Lorie, who was diagnosed as AD/HD in her senior year and has a history of chronic depression:

"Coaching has given me hope. Hope that I will really do what I say I am going to do. Since junior high school, I have felt hopeless and depressed because I couldn't stop the cycle of procrastinating. I would say to myself, 'This time it is going to be different, I am going to stay on top of all of my reading assignments,' but I never could, until I worked with my coach. This is the first time in my entire school career that I read all the assignments for my classes on time. I was able to do this because my coach and I defined bite-sized goals and I was accountable to her for completing them. I feel that this is the most important goal I have ever achieved in my life. Now, I have hope that I can continue to learn to do what I say I am going to do."

Jared, a part-time student with AD/HD, an expressive language disorder, and an anxiety disorder:

"I have always felt that there is greatness inside of me, but I lost any hope that this greatness would ever be realized. After years in special schools and lots of tutors and therapists, I feel I have finally figured out how to make my life better. While all those treatments helped me, I feel coaching has really helped me understand my disability and take action to change things. I used to work with tutors and teachers who would show me strategies and then I would go home and have no idea of how to apply those ideas. Coaching is more practical and personal. My coach and I figure out what strategies work for me and how to follow through on them. Also, I know that I am not alone. I email my coach every day to make sure I stay on track. She won't let me get off track or BS myself. I am changing and learning how to coach myself. Now, I believe I will actually use my greatness someday."

Stephanie, diagnosed with AD/HD in her senior year:

"I always felt negative about planning because I could never follow my plan. I hated calendars and day-planners because not only did I never use them, I would always lose them. Coaching has helped me create and use a planning process that works for me. I have learned to control time and not feel a victim, controlled by it. Basically, if I could reduce my thoughts about coaching to one thing, I'd say it is 'confidence.' I now have confidence that I really can do the things I want to do."

These students would all agree that coaching gives hope to the college student with AD/HD to learn to focus and control their attention and behavior in a way that no other intervention can. Since, coaching is not just about getting things done, but balance and self-awareness, as well, coaching has many long-term benefits. As a result of being coached, students begin to develop the tools for self-control and learn to coach themselves.

Benefits for professionals

There are also many benefits of using coaching with college students with AD/HD for the professionals doing the coaching. The following list summarizes some of these benefits.

- **Reduced stress during interactions with college students with AD/HD**

   At times, working with college students with AD/HD can be difficult and stressful for even the most seasoned professional. These students may be more likely than their peers to have difficulty staying focused during meetings, remembering appointments, and following through on plans. Coaching requires direct communication and the explicit discussion of the procedures for the relationship. Consequently, when faced with a perplexing situation, like how to handle the student's off-topic communication during a meeting or tendency to be late to an appointment, the coach openly discusses these issues with the student. Many times, problems are nipped in the bud because they have already been discussed in the initial meetings with students when the ground rules for meetings are being defined. If an issue arises that was not discussed previously, the relationship encourages asking the student, who is in the driver's seat, how to handle the situation. The coach is also encouraged to set boundaries and enforce them by direct com-munication with the student.

▪ Creativity is encouraged

Decision making about what to do and how to do it is ultimately the responsibility of the college student with AD/HD. As the student's partner, the coach is not solely responsible for knowing how to fix the problems the student presents. Instead, the coach sets the stage for creative problem-solving in which he or she provides suggestions and options, but isn't expected to know the answer. It is presumed that the student has the potential to create personalized solutions to the issues he or she faces and the coach unlocks the process of problem-solving by posing powerful questions. As a result, coaches report that students generate unique solutions to problems that the coach would never think of. The fact that there is no standardized curriculum or single solution is freeing to both the student and the coach. The dynamic coaching relationship allows for wonderful, creative solutions to be defined that are matched to each student's needs.

▪ Students are more likely to be invested in the process

Since students are in charge of what they do and how they choose to do it, they tend to be much more invested in the coaching relationship and in the plans that are developed. Therefore, coaching can be more rewarding than other more traditional teaching or tutoring relationships where the professional directs the sessions and the student's motivation and follow-through are sometimes deficient. Some students with AD/HD are diagnosed late in their school career and have little or no experience seeking help in such an intimate relationship. Many are relieved to discover that they are so involved in the process. Similarly, many students with AD/HD acknowledge being independent learners who prefer to learn from their own direct experience and not from the advice of others. Coaching is perfectly designed to match this style of learning.

Limitations of Coaching

In spite of all the benefits of coaching, it is not a cure all or panacea for college students with AD/HD. There are a number of limitations to using coaching as an intervention.

■ Students may not be ready for change

Sometimes students have been encouraged to get involved in a coaching relationship by their parents or the significant others in their lives because they want the student to change. In these instances, the truth may soon surface that the student isn't really ready to make changes in his or her life or to be held accountable by the coach. Coaching is not about talking about change or just talking about AD/HD. Coaching is designed to help the student take action and make the changes they want to make. When students don't follow through or they indicate that they would rather just talk than make plans for change, then it is time for the coach to again define what coaching is all about. No judgement needs to be made about the student, rather the coach and student may discover that a different form of intervention is needed. Perhaps the student really wants some education about AD/HD and needs to schedule meetings with the professional who did the evaluation or the physician who is prescribing medication or the college disability service provider. When the college disability service provider is also the coach, he or she may need to redefine the role and take off the hat of a coach and switch to the hat of the disability specialist, who can meet with the student to discuss AD/HD and its impact. Perhaps the student may discover that they came to the coach to please a parent and that this is not the optimal time for engaging a coach. It may be apparent that working with a therapist or counselor is the best thing at the moment, as the student deals with feelings that may be interfering with his or her functioning or ability to make changes.

■ **The professional may not be ready to be a coach**

Coaching is a very different intervention than tutoring, learning strategy instruction, therapy, or counseling. Therefore, coaching may require a major paradigm shift for the professional. Embracing the attitude that the person is whole, creative, resourceful, and not disabled or limited, may be very difficult for the professional who has spent years working from a deficit-centered approach to working with people. Letting go of old models of thinking, interpreting, and teaching can be very challenging. The professional must be ready to realize that he or she really doesn't know how to fix the student's problems and that the student is truly the expert. Therefore, the professional may not be ready or able to be a coach because of his or her beliefs and habit of taking charge and being the "expert."

■ **Coaching will not be enough**

The coaching interaction may help uncover the fact that other interventions are needed to complement the services of a coach. It may become apparent that the student truly has gaps in his or her skills in particular content areas, and that the services of a highly trained content tutor are needed. Perhaps the presence of weakness in the student's learning strategies may be uncovered, and the student may need to seek the support of a learning disabilities specialist to work on more basic academic strategies. Coaching may unmask the need for other consultants in a variety of areas, such as money management, personal organization, cooking, social skills, yoga, or stress management, to name a few. The need for counseling or therapy to deal with recurring emotional issues that may be interfering with the student's functioning may also be apparent as the coach and student evaluate progress. Additionally, the coaching relationship can assist the student in evaluating the need for medical interventions or the adjustment of currently prescribed medications. Coaching may also help determine that the student needs to seek out accommodations that "level the playing field" for the student's disability by contacting the disability services office on campus.

■ The demands of the college setting may exceed the student's skills

Even the best coaching relationship in the world cannot remove the problems that can be created when a student lacks the skills needed to succeed in a particular college setting. At times, a college student with AD/HD may have skill deficits or undiagnosed learning disabilities that are at odds with the highly competitive college climate he or she has selected. In these instances, coaching may help the student observe the mismatch that exists between academic or social expectations and his or her abilities. Coaching can provide a safe relationship in which to do this.

■ Getting training

The field of personal and professional coaching is relatively new, consequently, the training and competencies for coaches are currently being determined by the professional associations that are leading this field. Similarly, the field of AD/HD coaching is new and developing. Training procedures are evolving. Various organizations and individuals have developed training programs and certification processes, but it is up to the professional who is seeking training to be a consumer and to decide where and how to get training. To further complicate matters, there is currently no centralized or organized training available that is targeted to the unique issues that are faced when coaching college students with AD/HD.

▬ Anyone can say that they do coaching

For the parent who is seeking to employ a coach, the situation remains difficult, as well. Many professionals have added coaching to the list of services they offer, yet they may or may not have had any formal training in the strategies and skills that make coaching a unique service. Therefore, parents and young adults must be active consumers who collect information before agreeing to hire a professional who refers to him or herself as an AD/HD coach.

Conclusion

Coaching, very simply can be the "difference that makes a difference." Through the relationship with a coach, the student will be able to learn specific new strategies for setting goals and achieving objectives. He or she will be reminded of commitments made and of accomplishments forgotten. Through coaching, the student may feel moments of true redemption, without having to ask for forgiveness.

Just as in the field of athletics, the coach is there to encourage students to achieve their personal best, yet to accept any attempt, however halting and awkward, they make at trying. Sometimes the coach has to say, "Don't worry that you're going out there without a net. Right now, you're tangled up in a bunch of tight-rope!" Unlike parents, partners, or peers, the coach has absolutely no vested interest in the student's growth. Without ulterior motives or hidden agendas, the coach, nonetheless, secures and maintains a contract with the student.

By working with a coach, the student can come to a better understanding of his or her AD/HD, and clarify the impact that it has on daily life and academic success. With help, the student can learn how to recognize his learning style, and how to access and store information in a way that works for him. Coaching does not cure AD/HD or make the student less disabled. Instead, coaching can offer the student the opportunity to fall in love with learning again, and empower him to succeed.

PART
IV

RESOURCES

Resources

BOOKS

Barkley, R. A. (1997). *AD/HD and the Nature of Self-Control.* New York: Guilford Press.

Bramer, J. S. (1996). *Succeeding in College with Attention Deficit Disorders: Issues and Strategies for Students, Counselors and Educators.* Plantation, FL: Specialty Press.

Carson, R. (1983). *Taming Your Gremlin: A Guide to Enjoying Yourself.* New York: Harper Perennial.

Hallowell, E. M. and Ratey, J., (1994). *Driven to Distraction: Recognizing and Coping with Attention Deficit Disorder from Childhood to Adulthood.* New York: Pantheon Books.

Hartmann, T. and Bowman, J., (eds). (1996). *Think Fast! The ADD Experience.* Grass Valley, CA: Underwood Books.

Kelly, K. and Ramundo, P., (1995). *You Mean I'm Not Lazy, Stupid or Crazy?! A Self-help Book for Adults with Attention Deficit Disorder.* New York: Scribners.

Litt, Ann Selkowitz, (2000). *The College Student's Guide to Eating Well on Campus.* Bethesda, MD: Tulip Hill Press.

Nadeau, K. (1995). *A Comprehensive Guide to Attention Deficit Disorder in Adults: Research, Diagnosis, Treatment.* New York: Brunner/Mazel.

Nadeau, K. (1994). *College Survival Guide for Students with ADD or LD.* New York: Brunner/Mazel.

Quinn, P. O. (ed). (2000). *ADD and the College Student – Revised.* Washington, DC: Magination Press.

Quinn, P. O., and McCormick, A. (eds.). (1998). *Re-Thinking AD/HD: A Guide for Fostering Success in Students with AD/HD at the College Level.* Silver Spring, MD: Advantage Books.

Weiss, L. (1994). *The Attention Deficit Disorder in Adults Workbook.* Dallas: Taylor Publishing Company.

Wender, P. (1987). *The Hyperactive Child, Adolescent, and Adult: Attention Deficit Disorder through the Lifespan.* New York: Brunner/Mazel.

Whitworth, L., Kimsey-House, H, and Sandahl, P. (1998). *Coactive Coaching: New Skills for Coaching People Toward Success in Work and Life.* Palo Alto, CA: Davies-Black Publishing.

ARTICLES

Barkley, R. A. (1997, August). Update on a theory of AD/HD and its clinical implications. *The AD/HD Report,* 5:10-16.

Byron, J., and Parker, D. R (1997, Spring). Get on the bus: Responding to the needs of college students with AD/HD. *Post-secondary Disability Network News,* 30: 1-5.

Parker, D., (1998, Aug/Sept) Campuses report trends in college students with AD/HD. *Alert,* 22 (4): 42-44.

Journal of Postsecondary Education and Disability, (1995, Spring/Fall) Vol 11, Numbers 2 & 3, Special Issue on ADD.

PROFESSIONAL ASSOCIATIONS

Attention Deficit Disorder
ADDA—National Attention Deficit Disorder Association
847-432-ADDA/Fax 847-432-5874
www.add.org

AD-IN—Attention Deficit Information Network, Inc.
781-455-9895/fax 781-444-5466
www.addinfonetwork.com

CHADD—Children and Adults with Attention Deficit Disorder
800-233-4050 or 301-306-7070/Fax 301-306-7090
www.chadd.org

Learning Disabilities

LDA—Learning Disabilities Association of America
888-300-6710 or 412-341-1515/Fax 412-344-0224
www.ldanatl.org

NCLD—National Center for Learning Disabilities
888-575-7373 or 212-545-7510/Fax 212-545-9665
www.ncld.org

College Related

AHEAD—Association on Higher Education and Disability
617-287-3880/Fax 617-287-3881
www.ahead.org

Coaching

ADD Coaching
ACA—American Coaching Association
Director: Susan Sussman, M. Ed., ABDA, MCC
Phone/Fax 610-825-4505
www.Americoach.com

ICF—International Coaching Federation
1-888-ICF-3131 or 505-377-5937
www.coachfederation.org

COACH TRAINING

OFI—Optimal Functioning Institute
Director: Madeline Griffith-Haynie
423-524-9549/ Fax 423-524-1239
www.addcoach.com.

LCA—Limitbusters Coaching & Training, Inc.
Director: Eric Kohner
800-808-4476 or 626-351-9586/Fax 626-351-7703
www.limitbusters.com

ADDCA—ADD Coach Academy
Director: David Giwerc
518-482-3458/Fax 518-475-1992
www.addcoachacademy.com

Nancy Ratey, Ed.M., ABDA, MCC
781-237-3508
www.addbrain.com

Sandy Maynard, Director, Catalytic Coaching
202-884-0063
www.sandymaynard.com

Coach University
800-482-6224/Fax 800-329-5655
www.coachu.com

CTI—The Coaches Training Institute "Co-Active Coaching™"
800-691-6008 or 415-451-6000/Fax 415-460-6878
www.thecoaches.com

JOURNALS, NEWSLETTERS and PUBLICATIONS

ADD/LD and Related Issues
Focus
The Official Newsletter of the ADDA
www.add.org

The AD/HD Report
The Guilford Press
800-365-7006

The AD/HD Challenge
800-ADD-2322

Disability Compliance for Higher Education
LRP Publications
561-662-6520

ADDvance: A Magazine for Women with ADD
888-238-8588
www.addvance.com

ADDitude Magazine
www.additudemag.com

ALERT
Free newsletter from AHEAD
www.ahead.org

WORKBOOKS/MANUALS

Coaching Partners: An Alternative to Professional Coaching
    (A manual about Peer Coaching) Send $6 to the
    Adult A.D.D. Association, c/o Lisa Poast
    1225 E. Sunset Drive, Bellingham, WA 98226
    360-647-6681 dfhw32a@prodigy.com

A Resource Guide to Assistive Technology for Memory and Organization – 2nd edition, Published by:
Technology for Memory and Organization
718-444-0297

ADD Coach Sourcebook
Compiled by: Mary Jane Johnson
419-472-1990/Fax 419-472-7323

Personal Coaching
Facilitating Life Purpose: A Manual for Coaches
Developed by: Teri Belf, M.A., CAGS of SUN

VIDEOTAPES

Attention Deficit Disorder
AD/HD in Adults, Russell Barkley
(1998) [Videotape], The Guilford Press
800-233-9273

ADD and the College Student, P. O. Quinn
(1993) [Videotape], Pediatric Development Center
202-966-1561

Approaching College for Students with ADD, P.O.Quinn
(1993) [Videotape] Pediatric Development Center
202-966-1561

Outside-In: A Look at Adults with ADD
(1999) [Videotape], Family Today Inc.
Order from ADDA at www.add.org

Adults with ADD: Essential Information for ADD Adults
(1994) [Videotape], Child Management Inc., Producer
800-442-4453

ADD Coaching
Me, My ADD Coach and I
(2000) [Videotape] Videos for Change Production
1-877-5ADD-VIDEO

College Related
ADD: The Race Inside My Head
(1996) [Videotape] George Washington University, Producer
614-488-1174

Strategic Learning Videos: Dartmouth College
Contains a series of four videos (can be ordered individually or as a set)
800-257-5126

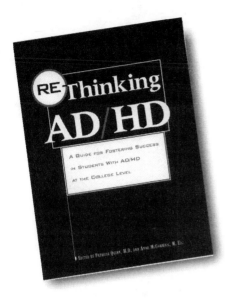